FLAT BELLY FIRM BUTT
IN 16 MINUTES

GET AN HOUR'S RESULTS IN 16 MINUTES

By MARIA BRILAKI

The advice contained within this book may be too strenuous for some people, and the reader should consult their health practitioner before engaging in the suggested activities. The information in this book is for educational purposes only. Neither the publisher nor the author is engaged in rendering professional advice or services to the individual reader. All matters regarding physical and mental health should be supervised by a health practitioner knowledgeable in treating that particular condition. Neither the author nor the publisher shall be liable or responsible for any loss, injury, or damage allegedly arising from any information or suggestion in this book. As with any diet or exercise program, if you experience any discomfort, stop immediately and consult your physician.

Designed by Maria Gratsia
Cover Picture: Maria Brilaki fitting in her tightest pants, performing the "Jeans Test" (see the "Track Your Progress" chapter).

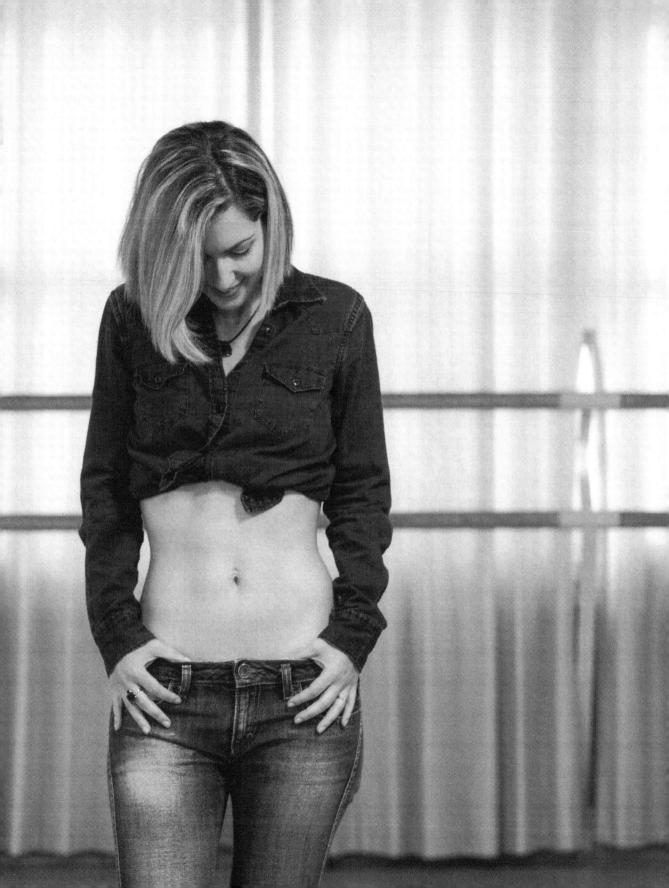

This book is dedicated to myself. Seriously. I know it may at first sound cocky, but we women too often opt for unnecessary humility instead of owning our accomplishments.

In this light, I want to dedicate this to myself: for developing FB16, my own perfect workout program; for keeping up with it, even when on vacation or while being seriously jet-lagged; for diligently writing this book; for the eight-hour exercise days it took to shoot the eight-week FB16 video program; and for inspiring others to look and feel great.

Just as I dedicate this book to myself, I want you to buy this book for you. To exercise for you, to praise yourself for everything that you achieve with it, and to own your success. My work is done. Now is the time for you to put your effort into this, and get the results you always wanted—in less time.

Everyone, let's do this. Are you ready?

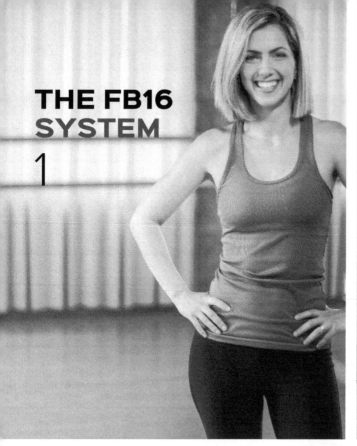

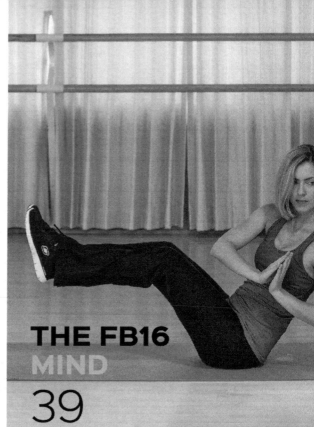

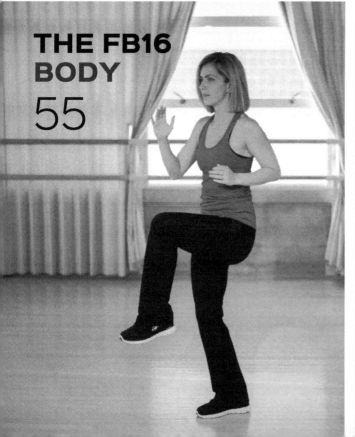

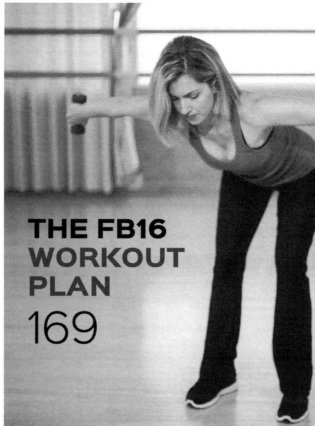

CONTENTS

X

FOREWORD

Welcome to the "Flat Belly, Firm Butt in 16 Minutes" workout program! Starting today, you can say good-bye to all the time-consuming workouts that ate up your time but gave you little in return. In the next four weeks, you'll be changing your fitness and getting visible results. From a flatter belly, tighter arms, and a straight back, to a lifted butt and nicely shaped legs, it'll all start happening as soon as you start the program.

If you've been disappointed because going to a 60-min yoga class, or running for 45 minutes on the treadmill doesn't seem to do much for your body, then FB16 is your kind of workout. It's short, it's effective, it's fun, and it gives you an hour's results in just 16 minutes. The next day after your workout, your muscles will feel the difference. Your body's fitness will rapidly go up. You'll find yourself having energy you never had before—not to mention all the flabbiness that will be replaced by neat, firm, non-jiggly matter. Your measuring tape will tell the story. Once you try FB16, you can never go back to spending hours on the treadmill.

Imagine this for a second. If you were to start exercising right now at this very moment, you'd be done in 16 minutes. Add another 10–15 minutes for your shower, and less than 30 minutes from now you'd have completed your workout, feel proud of yourself, smell nice, and would be wearing fresh, clean clothes.

Now compare this to going to the gym: 15 minutes to get there; one hour spent working out; another 15 minutes to come back; another 15 minutes to shower. Before you know it, almost two hours have gone by for the whole gym routine to be completed. That's almost an hour and a half longer compared to doing a 16-minute FB16 workout at home.

I know you'd much rather spend this time delivering at work, playing with your kids, watching a movie, or reading your favorite book. I do like exercise, but if I can get more with less, then count me in!

And there's more. The 16-minute solution of FB16 is so compelling that you'll find yourself having a hard time *not* doing it. You know all those workouts that you just can't do after a long day? Not the case with FB16.

FB16 doesn't require you to go to the gym and back. Bam—30 minutes were just saved. With FB16, you can just do it, right then and there. And you don't have to spend hours. You only need 16 minutes. You know you have 16 minutes. And most importantly, once you do it once, you know how effective those 16 minutes are. You know how they make your body feel and how they sculpt your physique. So not doing those 16 minutes that you know you can do and passing on those crazy benefits is just hard to do. FB16 is irresistible.

FB16 isn't one of the workouts that you'll do for a while and then put on the shelf and forget about it. Once you try it, it's hard to stop. It's almost addictive.

By following the four-week workout plan in this book:

- Up to five inches will be lost all over your body, including waist, hips, arms, thighs, and butt. You'll be admiring your new shape in the mirror.
- You'll get stronger. Whether you lift your baby with more ease or have more energy to wash the car, it'll start happening now!
- Your vitality will go up. You'll be keeping up with life better.
- You'll feel extremely proud of yourself and your confidence will increase.
- If you're already exercising, you'll be freeing about four hours a week by switching three of your normal workouts with FB16. How will you be spending those extra hours?
- You'll feel peace of mind that your fitness is in good hands. No need to worry about what to do or whether what you're doing is good enough— FB16 has you covered.

But let's set the right expectations here. FB16 will not make you super-model thin. Even though FB16 will give you the fastest results you could ever get from exercise, it's not a magic pill. The longer you stick to it, the more results you'll get.

FB16 is good for all levels, but it's also designed in such a way so that it'll keep challenging you as you're progressing.

Go to http://fitnessreloaded.com/fb16-book-resources/ to get:
- The bonus HD 16-minute workout that comes with this book.
- The Measurements Sheet to track your progress and the Four-week Workout Calendar.

Finally, bookmark this page: http://fitnessreloaded.com/interval-timer/. You'll be needing this interval timer to complete the fast-paced 16-minute workouts outlined in this book.

And for those of you who prefer doing video workouts, go to fitnessreloaded.com/fb16-home-workout/ to check out the FB16 eight-week video exercise program. It's a guided program that includes twelve full-length video FB16 workouts, eight weeks of e-mail guidance designed to keep you on track, a private Facebook group for support, and much more! Check it out.

Let's do it! FB16 might be short, fun, and effective, but the best workout in the world won't bring results until you actually do it! So now I want you to take a second and think about when you'd like to try your very first workout. Right now? Tomorrow? On Saturday at 6 p.m.? Put it on your calendar.

It's only 16 minutes, and if you follow the free video at http://fitnessreloaded.com/fb16-book-resources/, you don't need to read the whole book to get started. You can just do it, right now.

FB16 is not for the faint of heart, but it will transform your physique. No matter whether you've had good or bad experiences with exercise before, know that this is going to be different. No matter your starting point, I just wanted to say that I know you can do it. Let's get going.

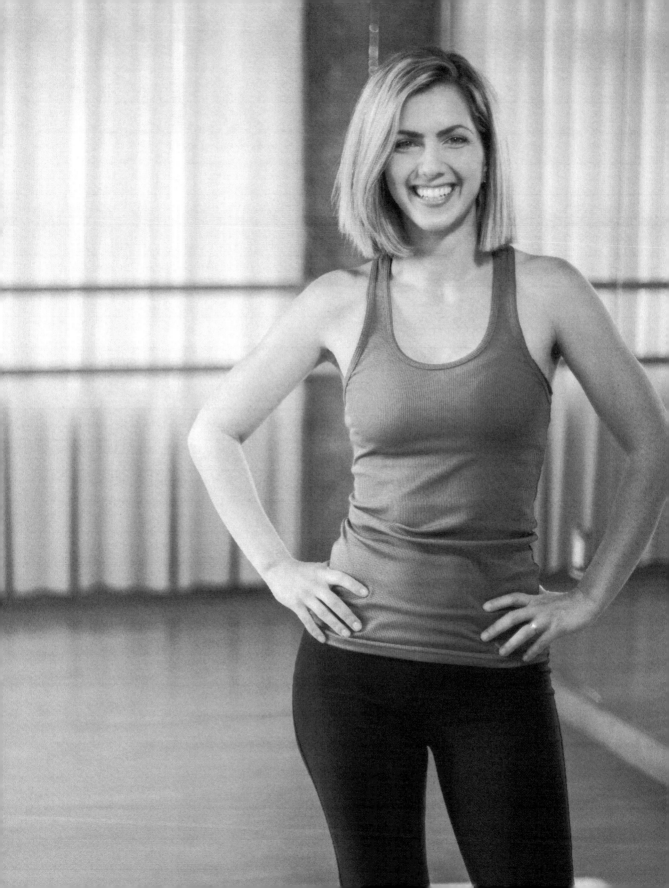

THE FB16 SYSTEM

It's All About Time

The number one reason people don't exercise is time. And who could blame them? A single spinning class or gym session can easily take two hours if you account for the time to drive there and back, and shower. If you're busy, have a career to advance, or have a family to raise—and more often than not, *both*— then it's really hard to find two hours out of your schedule multiple times per week to make it happen.

Yet even the people who do exercise often find exercise to be a chore. They'd much rather prefer that they could do less of it. Not that they don't necessarily like exercise. They love how exercise makes them look and feel. But with all the other things going on in their lives, it's very easy to feel like you could've been doing something *else* instead of exercise.

Now, FB16 is different. First off, it goes by really fast. Like lightning fast. It's only 16 minutes. It's not 16 minutes because you're compromising something; it's 16 minutes because you don't need more than that. Sixteen minutes of FB16 actually gets you more results than spending your normal hour at the gym. And you're going to experience this for yourself soon.

But it's not just fast; it's also found the sweet spot between being boring and being too unfamiliar. Let me explain. Have you ever done a workout that makes you do the same move again and again? Yes, that's boring. Have you also ever done a workout where all the exercises were brand new to you? So new that it was hard for you to follow as you had to figure out all those differ-ent new moves? My first time in a yoga class was like that-way too unfamiliar. In FB16, I feel I've hit the sweet spot. When I asked the original group of people who did the eight-week video program about this, here's what they said.

"Using a 1–10 scale, how would you rate this program in terms of exercise variety? Why?"

- "10. There were a lot of exercises I've never done, which was surprising. But it also had enough repetition that I wasn't lost and feeling like every time I had to learn something new."
- "I agree with Jessica: 10. It also meant that I never got bored or conquered all; there's always a challenge, an exercise you can do better, like sideways plank!"
- "10. It was a great balance of very difficult exercises and more accessible exercises. It will be a while before I can still perfect every move."
- "Oh my gosh, variety is your specialty! I give you a flat out 10! You move from one exercise to another without being repetitive in any of the workout sets. They each graduate in intensity and only are repeated one time; not a single one of your workout sets was a repeat of the other… instead, they each built upon one another."
- "I would say a 10 as it worked every part of the body and you were never bored doing the same thing over and over. Congrats to you, Maria, for setting the program up so well…."
- "I give it a whole-hearted 10! I LOVED these exercises! All of them! And this comes from someone who never managed to like working out."
- "I rate it a very high 10 also. As a 'home exercise DVD junkie,' I've tried a lot. Some I liked, some I couldn't do. For me, I prefer a faster pace (I get bored easily), but some of the 'dance' DVDs are just too complicated to keep up with. And once they go beyond 20 minutes or so, I no longer have enough time to devote to it. This was fast, challenging, achievable, and new. All those DVDs…and you had really good moves I've never seen before!"

Okay, let me just stop here with all the 10 ratings. Needless to say, 100% of the people gave the eight-week video program a 10! So, yes, you can feel confident this is not a program that will bore you.

This is also not a program that you do just to "lose weight" or "burn fat." The way you exercise is the way you build your body. And you want to build your body the right way, not haphazardly. That's why I seek to create a deeper change than just burning fat. I want you to walk straighter. Stand taller. Feel more confident. Be less scared to push yourself to uncharted territories. Deeply understand the right form of each exercise so that you feel confident you do it right—and don't hurt yourself either. This program is not about mindlessly doing each exercise, hoping that you're burning calories. This is about feeling each exercise, feeling the burn, pushing through it, and finishing each workout feeling you became a bit better than 16 minutes earlier when you started it.

FB16 is definitely not about perfection. It's about progress. I don't care how many repetitions you do. I don't care if you need to stop because you're out of breath. I don't care how low you go on squats. I don't care if your balance is unstable. What I care about is that you give it your all—for 16 minutes. That's all I ask. And I know that if you do that, with every workout you'll get better, stronger, fitter, and leaner. And that's enough. Before you know it, others will be commenting about it. Your energy levels will be higher. You will be sleeping better at night. Your lab results will improve. And you will need to get different pants—smaller ones.

Why I Created FB16

"Results-focused" vs. "easy-going" exercise

There's "results-focused" exercise, and then there's "easy-going" exercise. "Results-focused" exercise is when you're pushing yourself. You don't cheat. You don't try to do less repetitions, lift lower weights, or run shorter distances. You take it to the next level. That's the type of exercise that sculpts your physique: your arms get leaner, your butt tighter, your abs flatter. Dress sizes drop, and inches are lost. Your strength and endurance go up, and suddenly you realize you no longer get as tired as you used to. That's exactly what "results-focused" exercise does for you.

"Easy-going" exercise is usually less demanding. It's the type of exercise where you don't need to push yourself to make it happen. It's when you lift what you've always lifted (making small incremental changes at best), when you run the route that feels like second nature to you, or when you go for a walk to get your daily 30 minutes in. It feels good to get moving, and with every workout you add days to your life, but you're not really changing the shape of your body. With time, most workouts that start as "results-focused" exercise inevitably transition into "easy-going" exercise.

This book is about "results-focused" exercise. Of course, I'm by no means against "easy-going" exercise. On the contrary, I think we desperately need more of it in our lives. Most of us sit way too much, often spending eight or ten hours a day on a chair or sofa. Sitting has dramatic effects on our health and longevity. It's no coincidence that one of the world's longest-lived populations, the people in Ikaria, an island in Greece, do not focus on "results-focused" exercise. They do a lot of "easy-going" exercise and a small amount of "results-focused" exercise. They farm and perform gardening tasks. They walk. They swim. And they live to be 100 or more.

I firmly believe that the optimal "amount" of exercise to live healthy and vital and age to be 100 or more includes mostly "easy-going" exercise and a small amount of "results-focused" exercise. "Results-focused" exercise makes you look your best and takes your muscles and endurance to the next level.

"Easy-going" exercise is like a lubricant you apply to your joints, the oil you put into your engine. Your body needs this daily to function properly.

Now, the lines between "results-focused" and "easy-going" exercise can be blurry sometimes. I still remember years ago watching a 100-year-old+ man on Greek TV. He said that every day he'd walk to the woods and cut firewood with his axe. He'd then use the logs to warm his house in the winter.

I saw this 100-year-old man on TV working the huge axe and cutting the wood, and I kept thinking: "I'm in my twenties, but I'm not as strong as this 100-year-old grandpa! There's no way I could do that for 15 minutes let alone for hours every day!"

Now does wood-cutting count as "results-focused" or as "easy-going" exercise? Maybe he was so used to the axe that even wood-cutting counted as "easy-going" exercise. But I think it was a combination. Just like the people of Ikaria who walk a lot and also do multiple hardcore gardening and farming jobs, this guy spent a good chunk of his day walking, but he'd also work the axe. And the axe kept him in top shape.

How I met High Intensity Interval Training (HIIT)

After I gained weight as a graduate student at Stanford engineering, I decided I'd make healthy living a priority. Since then, I've been moving my body almost religiously five times a week. By "moving" I refer to a combination of "results-focused" and "easy-going" exercise: from weight lifting and cardio at the gym, to yoga and pilates classes, to brisk walking, to barre-type and High Intensity Interval Training at-home DVDs.

My attempts to find the perfect workout started at the gym. With time I began switching up my gym routine. I went from doing five weight lifting exercises to seven or nine, and then after a while went back to three or five—but added 15 minutes of stretching and 25 minutes of cardio. None of these changes produced any significant difference on my body, but at the time, I didn't care that much about results. I was content with enjoying myself when working out.

You see, my number one goal was—and is—to live a long life. "Easy-going" exercise is just what you need to make it happen. For longevity, you don't need to exert yourself too much—but you do need to keep moving! Even though I didn't revel in just maintaining my fitness and only making incremental improvements, I was okay with my workout schedule. Maybe I didn't bother with the absence of results, because I just didn't know what was possible. Most importantly, I didn't know that I could enjoy myself just as much, and get amazing results as well. Who said you have to sacrifice joy for results?

And then I discovered HIIT—High Intensity Interval Training. When doing interval training you alternate between very intense short bursts of exercise and rest. HIIT posed a different type of challenge, and I wanted to explore it more. I soon replaced a weekly 60-minute-long gym workout with a (legs-focused) 16-minute HIIT workout. I felt a bit guilty for exercising "less," but at the same time I enjoyed being done in 16 minutes rather than the normal hour and a half of going to the gym and back.

A month later I noticed something different about my legs. They were leaner. There was definition that didn't exist before. They had changed shape a bit. They were less of an inverted triangle, as they were narrower at the hip level than they used to be. But why? What had changed?

And then it dawned on me. HIIT was the only thing that had changed. I thought I was slacking by only doing a 16-minute HIIT workout, but it seemed that this workout produced far more effective results than my normal 60-minute gym session.

I was impressed! I had never seen results that fast. And the passion for changing my physique while getting stronger and fitter came back.

Workouts either take too much time or give too little results

The accidental results rekindled my passion for resculpting and redefining my body. And that's how I decided I had to go back to doing more "results-focused" exercise. Yet going to the gym and lifting more wouldn't give me the fast results I had just experienced. Plus, most HIIT workouts were boring and repetitive, suggesting I do the same few exercises over and over again until time was up. Enjoying my workout was still number one on my requirements list, and having fun was a criterion I had no intention of giving up.

So if going to the gym was not going to cut it, then what would? I tried yoga and pilates classes, but they were not really bringing accelerated results. Plus they were exactly that: classes. I had to be at the studio at a specific time and date. This didn't work very well for my free-spirited soul.

It was no accident that I had made brisk walking a habit in just a few months. I went from walking to the next block and back to four or five miles at a time. Whenever my body felt stiff, I could put my headphones on and go. I loved the instant availability of walking. But walking qualifies as "easy-going" exercise, not as "results-focused."

Finally, I started experimenting more and more with home workout DVDs. My experience was mixed. Some teachers I really liked, some others not so much. Some DVDs I'd do again and again, and some others I couldn't even finish. Some exercises would make me sore, some would push me to the limit, and some were too easy. Some workouts would be 50 minutes long or more, others would be broken into 10-minute segments, and others would take me around 30 minutes to complete.

Unlike going to yoga or pilates classes, working out at home comes easier to me. Just like walking, I can work out at home whenever I want to. Is it a Saturday morning and I have 45 minutes available? Pop in a DVD and get moving! Is it 11 p.m. at night? Just do it. Nothing can stop me from exercising at my own house. Not the weather or anything else.

But my home DVDs experience was varied. The difficult 30-minute HIIT workouts would definitely give me results. I had never seen my arms so well shaped! But there was a problem. I needed my husband to put them on, otherwise I'd never do them on my own. I found them repetitive, too strenuous, and less efficient than I liked, often mixing "good" exercises with "filler exercises" (i.e., exercises that have little impact on the body by only working one or two muscles max or by being too easy).

The ballet, pilates, or yoga-type DVDs sat well with me. I enjoyed doing them on cold winter nights or sleepy Saturday mornings, but those were also not the workouts that would give me the results I was looking for.

And then there was this other DVD—the one I'd do again and again. It didn't give me the results of HIIT, but it was still pushing me. Lots of exercise variety, upbeat instructors, 20 minutes long, fun music—that was a workout I was looking forward to.

The problem? My passion for results was not satisfied. I knew that a HIIT workout would give me better and faster body definition and fitness. My body was getting used to the new moves way too fast. Sooner rather than later, this DVD went from "results-focused" to "easy-going" exercise.

I had yet to find a fun home workout that would give me the real results I was looking for—a workout that I'd want to do again and again, and that would keep me challenged as my fitness level increased.

The elements of the perfect workout

Through trial and error, my "perfect workout" preferences were getting clearer and clearer. Why was I doing some DVDs repeatedly, while some others I'd only do a couple of times? Why would I do difficult HIIT workouts together with my husband, but I'd almost never do them on my own? And most importantly, what would the "perfect" workout be for me? What would a workout need to have to make me want to do it again and again and give me results at the same time? The elements of the "perfect" workout started emerging:

- The perfect workout is instantly available. You don't need to be somewhere at a specific time and date to do it. It's just there for you.
- The perfect workout is effective. Multiple workouts have "effective" exercises out there, but they combine them with so many "filler" ones. You end up getting too little in return for your efforts. Other workouts are full of breaks, unnecessarily wasting your time. The perfect workout, though, is "condensed": it gets a lot done in a short amount of time. It doesn't waste two or three minutes between exercises. It doesn't let you cheat by doing less than what you're capable of. The perfect workout pushes you further and further.
- The perfect workout hits the "variety sweet spot." You don't do the same movement again and again, repetition after repetition, until seven minutes later your muscles can't take it anymore. You don't repeat a round

of exercises four or five times. At the same time, you don't do completely different exercises each time, and hence avoid getting lost and feeling frustrated because of the learning curve. Instead, the perfect workout has the perfect combo between new and old exercises.

- The perfect workout works the whole body. It's not just about abs, or arms, or legs. It's not about strength training or cardio. It's about everything.

- And finally, the perfect workout is fun. It's not boring, it does not include you looking at the clock and sighing as you realize that you've only done the first ten minutes. It does not make you do the same, boring moves for an hour. Instead, it makes you feel like times passes fast! Before you know it, it's already over! You had such a good time, you didn't even notice how fast time went by!

Since the "perfect workout" was not yet out there, I decided I had to scratch my own itch. These are exactly the criteria that I used to create the "Flat Belly, Firm Butt in 16 minutes" eight-week video workout program, and that's how this book was born. FB16 is my own perfect workout and I'm delighted to be sharing it with you.

The Foundation: High Intensity Interval Training

FB16 is based on the principles of High Intensity Interval Training (HIIT). When performing HIIT, you're alternating between intense bursts of exercise and short rest periods. HIIT workouts normally last between four and 30 minutes.

But what is an intense workout? An intense workout usually pushes your heart rate to 75% or more of its maximum. Now, how do you find your maximum heart rate (MHR)? Subtract your age from 220. E.g., if you're 30 years old, your MHR is 190. So if you're doing High Intensity Training at 75% of your heart rate, that would give you 142.5 beats per minute. If you did low intensity exercise at 60% of your MHR, then you'd get 114 beats per minute. You see now how your heart beats faster when you're doing more intense exercise.

Now, let's set the math aside and talk results. As mentioned before, when I first switched one of my normal hour-long workouts with a legs-focused 16-minute HIIT one, I felt as if I was slacking and doing less. A month later, I was wondering what happened to my legs. Why were they leaner? I was noticing definition that I had never seen before. I would poke them with my finger, and I'd feel that they were stronger. And that's when it hit me: It was HIIT! Even though I was only doing it once a week, and even though I thought I was cheating because I was only exercising a quarter of an hour, my body was responding extremely well to it. I was both surprised and impressed.

But my experience is not a solo incident. It has scientifically been proven that HIIT gets you extremely fast results. From health benefits, to improved aerobic capacity, muscle growth, and fat loss, studies have indicated that HIIT is surprisingly effective. Many studies even indicate that HIIT doesn't just get you fast results, it gets you results faster than doing longer workouts. Work out less, get more results. Amazing, right? Let's dive in.

The fitness metric

Before we start discussing how studies indicate that HIIT may be superior to moderate exercise, let me explain the terminology first. VO2 max (also maximal oxygen consumption, maximal oxygen uptake, peak oxygen uptake, or maximal aerobic capacity) is the maximum rate of oxygen consumption as measured during incremental exercise, most typically on a treadmill.

This is the single best measure of fitness and aerobic endurance, and that's why it's extremely common to find it in studies. Scientists use it to measure whether, and if yes how much, the method they are testing is increasing the fitness level of the participants.

Is HIIT more effective than moderate exercise for losing fat?

You may think you need to slave at the gym on the treadmill, the stationary bike, or the elliptical. But this might not be the optimal way to lose fat. Trapp et al.[1] conducted a High Intensity program for 15 weeks with three weekly 20-minute HIIT sessions in young women. HIIT consisted of an eight-second sprint followed by 12 seconds of low intensity cycling. Another group of women carried out an aerobic cycling protocol that consisted of steady state cycling at 60% VO2 max for 40 minutes. Results showed that women in the 20-minute HIIT group lost significantly more fat (2.5 kg or 5.5 lb.) than those in the 40-minute steady state aerobic exercise program. I call this efficiency, don't you? And this is only the beginning.

HIIT burns more calories once exercise is over

The post-exercise period is called "EPOC", which stands for excess post-exercise oxygen consumption. This two-hour period is when the body is restoring itself to pre-exercise levels, and hence using more energy. Because high intensity training is harder exercise than moderate training, it requires more energy from the body, leading to a six to 15% higher calorie burn.[2]

Now, don't get too hung up on this. EPOC calorie burn is very little compared to the calories burned during your workout, so even if you burn 15% more calories during the EPOC period, this is still too small to help get rid of your

1 Trapp EG, Chisholm DJ, Freund J, Boutcher SH. The effects of high-intensity intermittent exercise training on fat loss and fasting insulin levels of young women. International Journal of Obesity. 2008;32(4):684–691
2 Information on High Intensity Interval Training, American College of Sport Medicine, 2014

saddlebags. EPOC is a nice add-on though. That's why you might hear about it either online or in magazines.

But how much do you really need to exercise to get results?

Professor Martin Gibala from the Department of Kinesiology at McMaster University got digging. He found that as little as seven minutes of HIIT is enough to produce results. Seven minutes?! Impressive, huh?

Yet he also said this may not be safe for the average person. Unless you are an athlete, it's hard to push to your maximum continuously for seven minutes. So if pushing to your max for seven continuous minutes is not possible, then how can you still get the benefits of intense exercise?

Gibala and his collaborators started looking at different forms of High Intensity Interval Training. A model they experimented with was one minute of hard exercise followed by one minute of rest, repeated 10 times. That gives us a total of 10 minutes of pure exercise in a span of 20 minutes. Repeated just three times a week, this model gives a mere 60 minutes a week—significantly less than the common recommendations of 150 minutes a week.

Apparently, even 60 minutes a week is enough to bring results. In a type 2 diabetes study[3] he performed, just two weeks of following this model gave participants a significant drop in their blood sugar levels. "Basically, their heart becomes a better, stronger pump, your blood vessels get more elastic and that's helpful to allow blood and oxygen to flow. And your muscles get better at using that oxygen, so you feel less tired," Gibala explained.[4]

In just two weeks and in just 60 minutes of exercise a week Gibala's study indicates that you don't need to exercise for 150 minutes in order to get significant health benefits.

HIIT might be the fastest way to increase your fitness

Okay, so we know HIIT is beneficial to our bodies, but the real question here

3 Little JP, Gillen JB, Gibala MJ, et al. Low-volume high-intensity interval training reduces hyperglycemia and increases muscle mitochondrial capacity in patients with type 2 diabetes. J Appl Physiol. 2011 Dec;111(6):1554-60.
4 As reported to CTV Toronto's Pauline Chan.

is, does HIIT improve your fitness level faster than moderate exercise? Gibala et al. studied the effects of sprint-interval training versus high volume endurance training.[5] Sprint interval training is a type of high intensity training where people specifically perform sprints as their main form of exercise. The authors studied 16 men in total, eight in each one of the two groups. Both groups worked out six times a week for a total of two weeks.

The HIIT group performed four to six repeats of 30-second "all out" cycling at ~250% V_{O_2peak} with four-minute recovery. The endurance group did 90–120 minutes of continuous cycling at ~65% V_{O_2peak}. Overall, the HIIT group worked out for 2.5 hours, while the endurance group devoted 10.5 hours. The authors found that six sessions of either low volume sprint-interval training or traditional high volume endurance training induced similar improvements in muscle oxidative capacity, muscle buffering capacity, and exercise performance. In other words, 2.5 hours of high-intensity exercise gives you the same results as 10.5 hours of exercise. The numbers here speak for themselves.

But what about HIIT's health benefits? Let's start from the heart

No matter who you are, physical exercise is taxing on the heart. Having coronary heart and artery disease makes it crucial to engage in aerobic activity. But HIIT brings good news: If you have heart complications and are ready to take up a cardio method, interval training might actually be a better choice over traditional endurance training.[6] Interval training brings no increasing risk but similar or even greater max benefits than endurance training.

A 2004 study from the European Journal of Preventive Cardiology evaluated the effects of high intensity to moderate intensity aerobics (three times a week, ten weeks) in cardiac patients. The authors' concluding remarks:

"High intensity aerobic interval exercise is superior to moderate exercise for increasing V_{O_2peak}...and may be useful in designing effective training pro-

5 Gibala M, Little J, Van Essen M, et al. Short-term sprint interval versus traditional endurance training: similar initial adaptations in human skeletal muscle and exercise performance. The Journal of Physiology. 2006;575: 901-911.
6 Rognmo O, Hetland E, Helgerud J, et al. High intensity aerobic interval exercise is superior to moderate intensity exercise for increasing aerobic capacity in patients with coronary artery disease. Eur J Cardiovasc Prev Rehab. 2004;11(3):216-222.

grammes for improved health in the future."[7] A big win for interval training!

And there are more heart-loving indications that interval training produces similar or even better results in less time. With age comes increased risk of heart failure. Twenty-seven elderly patients (>70 years) that survived a heart attack or other form of heart failure were randomized into two groups; one that did interval training at 95% peak heart rate, and one that did moderate continuous training at 70% peak heart rate. Both trainings were conducted three times per week for 12 weeks. The interval training group noted *better* improvement at their cardiovascular system function compared to the moderate continuous training group.[8] Again, another study compared the effects of interval training vs. moderate continuous training but with coronary artery bypass grafting patients. Results indicated that compared to moderate continuous training, interval training enhances both long-term oxygen uptake and present and future quality of life.[9]

Any form of exercise is good for our health, but it seems that interval training must take a special place in our heart, and for a good reason.

HIIT lowers your blood pressure

Blood pressure is an important factor monitored in hypertension screenings. So it begs the question: Between interval training, moderate intensity aerobics or strength training, which one would lower blood pressure most? Both aerobic exercises (interval training and moderate intensity) decreased systolic blood pressure, but interval training, rather than moderate aerobic exercise, kept it significantly lowered for much longer.[10] It seems that pushing yourself to the next level brings longer lasting results.

---

7 Ibid.
8 Wisløff U, Støylen A, Loennechen JP, et al. Superior cardiovascular effect of aerobic interval training versus moderate continuous training in heart failure patients: a randomized study. Circulation. 2007;115(24):3086-3094.
9 Moholdt TT, Amundsen BH, Rustad LA, et al. Aerobic interval training versus continuous moderate exercise after coronary artery bypass surgery: a randomized study of cardiovascular effects and quality of life. Am Heart J. 2009;158(6):1031–1037.
10 Schjerve IE, Tyldum GA, Tjønna AE, et al. Both aerobic endurance and strength training programmes improve cardiovascular health in obese adults. Clin Sci (Lond). 2008;115(9):283–293.

More studies showing HIIT to be superior to moderate exercise

Aerobic training itself helps manage metabolic syndrome, a cluster of health problems that increase the risk for cardiovascular disease, diabetes, and stroke. And yes, individuals with metabolic syndrome are three times more likely to die of heart disease than their healthy counterparts. What is in doubt is what type of aerobic training helps the best.

Tjonna et al. had 32 metabolic syndrome patients split into two groups (continuous and interval training) to train three times a week for 16 weeks doing equal volumes of exercise. Interval training was superior to continuous training in regulating insulin in fat and skeletal muscle, reducing blood glucose, and creating less fatty tissue.[11] Continuing on, another metabolic syndrome study (using rats and the rat model) had similar results to Tjonna et al. but with further findings of increased maximal oxygen uptake, reduced hypertension, and lowered LDL cholesterol, aka "bad cholesterol," levels. The study concluded that "exercise training reduces the impact of the metabolic syndrome and that the magnitude of the effect depends on exercise intensity."[12] In other words, exercising at an intense—rather than moderate—pace gives higher health benefits.

When it comes to health, these studies indicate that interval training may be a promising alternative to traditional continuous endurance training. The scientific community is gradually recognizing that we may indeed be able to get more with less. I can't wait to see what the community will have discovered a few years from now when more studies will be completed comparing the health benefits of these two forms of exercise.

HIIT seems promising, but isn't it too intense? Am I going to hate it?

No! You might even like it. After all, exercise is not just about what it does to our body. It's also about what it does to our mood and happiness. And surprising-

---

11 Tjonna AE, Lee SJ, Rognmo O, et al. Aerobic interval training versus continuous moderate exercise as a treatment for the metabolic syndrome: a pilot study. Circulation. 2008;118(4):346-54.
12 Haram PM, Kemi OJ, Lee SJ, et al. Aerobic interval training vs. continuous moderate exercise in the metabolic syndrome of rats artificially selected for low aerobic capacity. Cardiovasc Res. 2009;81(4):723-32.

ly, even though HIIT is tiring, that doesn't reduce the pleasure derived from it. Yes, you read that right—pleasure.

In their article, Bartlett et al. said that despite higher ratings of perceived exertion, "high-intensity interval running is perceived to be more enjoyable than moderate-intensity continuous exercise."[13] Another study reported that even though High Intensity Training was selected as more tiring, it still got an overall enjoyment level equal to the one of continuous exercise.[14]

Again, you get more but without feeling like it sucks. So if that was a concern, well, you can cross that out now. Now, let's talk weight loss.

13 Bartlett JD, Close GL, MacLaren DP, et al. High-intensity interval running is perceived to be more enjoyable than moderate-intensity continuous exercise: implications for exercise adherence. J Sports Sci. 2011;29(6):547-53.
14 Oliveira BRR, Slama FA, Deslandes AC, et al. Continuous and High-Intensity Interval Training: Which Promotes Higher Pleasure? PLoS One. 2013;8(11):e79965.

How Much Do I Really Need to Exercise to Lose Weight?

I'm not here to sell you hype. I know HIIT is hot and trendy now (and as shown before for a good reason), but I do want you to have a well-rounded perspective about exactly what it takes to lose weight—if that's your goal.

First, let me address the elephant in the room. For most people, eighty percent of weight loss will come from following a better diet. It's extremely hard to out-exercise a bad diet. A 130-pound marathon runner will only burn 2,224 calories during a marathon[15]—less than the 3,500 calories needed to burn a pound. So you're effectively burning 63% of a pound by running a 26.2-mile course! That's how much exercise it takes to lose weight, and that's why exercise is usually only 20% of weight loss.

Of course, you *can* make exercise be 80% of weight loss. But that would require you to exercise for hours and hours every day (or accept you'll lose weight very slowly). For most people, it's much easier to eat less calories than to devote all this time burning all the calories they've consumed. And that's how the 80-20 ratio comes out.

So what can exercise really do for you? Here's my own experience. Exercise has completely reshaped my body. I stand taller. My shoulders look much better. My butt is firmer. My abs are just awesome. My thighs have less of a triangular shape (still narrow at knee level but much less expanded on my upper thighs). I can be firm or I can be flabby. I choose firm.

And it's not just about looks. My endurance is much higher. I get less tired when going for walks or hikes. I feel better, as exercise is my daily stress-buster. Not to mention all the diseases that I probably won't get just because I'm protecting myself by regularly exercising. Oh, and what about living longer? Even 15 minutes of recreational exercise a day can lead to living three years longer.[16]

15 Cleveland Clinic Center for Consumer Health,
http://www.clevelandclinic.org/health/interactive/calories.asp
16 Wen CP, Wai JP, Tsai MK, et al. Minimum amount of physical activity for reduced mortality and extended life expectancy: a prospective cohort study. Lancet. 2011;378(9798):1244-53.

I don't know about you, but I'm totally sold! Exercise is precious! My life would just not be the same without it, and I know that if you exercise too you must feel the same way.

Last but not least, the 20% component of exercise to weight loss does have a significant effect on the body. I can eat the equivalent of a small piece of cake on the days when I exercise without gaining more weight. I'm not saying I eat cake every time I exercise—I just want to make a point: When you exercise, you can eat more. Even yummy food. Guilt-free.

Okay, so we've established how exercise is benefiting you. But what should you do if your primary goal is weight loss? High intensity exercise is obviously more effective than moderate intensity. It's only natural to burn more calories in 15 minutes of high intensity exercise vs. 15 minutes of moderate intensity exercise. So yes, if you could work out for 40 minutes continuously at a high intensity exercise mode, you'd burn many more calories than if you went for a 60-minute brisk walk. But can you really do 40 continuous minutes of high intensity exercise?

Not really. And that's why I think that if you're optimizing for weight loss, you need to strategically combine moderate- with high-intensity exercise, or else, "results-focused" and "easy-going" exercise. You'll do the high-intensity part to rapidly improve your endurance and muscle growth, developing that strong and lean body you crave. And then you'll follow up with the moderate-intensity part to help boost your calorie burn.

For example, you could do a 16-minute FB16 workout and then follow up with 30 minutes of brisk walking. You get a significant caloric burn by exercising for 45+ minutes in addition to all the rapid results that come from high intensity training. This is indeed the best of both worlds.

Now, if you don't need to lose weight, you obviously don't have to go for walks. But let me preach a bit here. Most of us spend the day sitting. We have sedentary jobs. We sit and slouch. Sitting has now been declared the smoking of our generation, and it rapidly increases our mortality risk.[17] Even if you don't

---

17 Van der Ploeg HP, Chey T, Korda RJ, et al. Sitting Time and All-Cause Mortality Risk in 222 497 Australian Adults. Arch Intern Med. 2012;172(6):494-500.

want to lose weight, I am a big advocate of reducing sitting time. And going for walks, or even having meetings while walking, is a great way to stand up and let yourself move.

And no, exercising is not enough to prevent the mortality risks of sitting. Just like exercising doesn't protect you from the risks of lung cancer that come from smoking, it is similar with sitting. Sitting for eight hours a day or more is taking its toll even if you exercise. So the more you move, the better.

How The FB16 Exercises Were Selected

All the exercises chosen for the FB16 program had to qualify themselves through the "efficient and effective" rule. You see, we're inundated with exercises—exercises for our abs, butt, legs, arms, etc. But not all exercises are made equal. Some exercises are just more effective than others. Some exercises get you the same results but in less time. With FB16, you can sleep at night without worry. You know you're getting the very best exercise can offer you. Every exercise included in FB16 was strategically selected as an "efficient and effective" exercise. There are no "filler" exercises here. You're not wasting your time.

To abide by the "efficient and effective" rule and exercise your whole body, the hand-picked exercises of FB16 come from a variety of sources and serve different purposes.

Isometric exercises

Isometrics make you hold the same pose for a long time. Their beauty is not just that they work your muscles, but that often, in order to help you keep your balance and stabilize yourself, they make you use multiple tiny muscles other than the primary muscles being worked. These muscles would otherwise not be put to work if it were not for isometrics.

Bodyweight exercises

FB16 is mainly comprised of bodyweight exercises, i.e., exercises that only use your body's own weight to work your muscles. I love bodyweight exercises because they help you function better in every-day life. Think about it: you walk around all day carrying your own weight; you squat down to pick something from the floor, again carrying your own weight. Training with bodyweight exercises will make every-day life movements much easier, and will give you some protection against common injuries that happen when you accidentally do a move you shouldn't have done.

Not only are they immensely effective, but they're also convenient. You can do them anytime, anywhere. Combine them with the short, 16-minute duration and you know you have a winner, a workout you can take with you wherever you are.

Weight-bearing exercises
In FB16, we're also incorporating weights, mostly dumbbells. Unlike other exercise programs that "pick a side" on the bodyweight vs. weightlifting debate, in FB16, we pick the best of what every type of training has to offer. So when bodyweight exercises help your muscles grow the most, then bodyweight exercises we'll do. But if it's weightlifting exercises that bring the best results, then weights we'll lift. I've found that especially when it comes to arms and shoulders, using weights can really bring you the extra definition you need faster than if you were to just try to get the same effect with bodyweight exercises. And that's why for our upper body workouts, we're also using dumbbells.

And that's how FB16 builds lean muscle mass, which is exactly what you're looking for if you want to see definition in your body. Losing fat alone doesn't give you definition; at best, you'll be skinny-flabby. It's exercise that'll build up your body, make you stronger, remove the jiggly parts, and replace them with firm muscle tissue. And that's how your butt stops being saggy or "wavy" and starts being lifted and firm.

Cardio component
Do you think you need a treadmill to do cardiovascular exercise? No you don't. FB16 not only includes cardio exercises, but by pushing you to fit in as many repetitions as possible through the HIIT regimen, it takes cardio to the next level. The whole FB16 workout will actually get your heart rate up, even when you're not doing traditional cardio exercises.

Stretching exercises
I love stretching. I do 15 minutes of stretching after every workout. Why? Because I love improving my flexibility. But in FB16, stretching is recommended, not mandatory. Why? Because stretching is not necessary to get you fast results. Yes, it does help you avoid soreness, and it does lengthen your muscles;

it's also beneficial for your posture. But again, it's not necessary for a flat belly and a firm butt. You can get a flat belly and a firm butt without stretching. And since we want to be time-efficient, I leave stretching up to your judgment.

If you're not hard-pressed on time, spend two to three minutes at the end of each workout to stretch your muscles. Giving yourself some time to cool down after an intense workout and giving your muscles the opportunity to "unwind" will make you feel so much better afterwards, plus you may feel less sore the day after.

From now on, don't spend your time worrying about your fitness. FB16 will take care of that. You're free to use your mind to advance in your career or to play with your family—leave fitness on FB16. You won't be disappointed.

The FB16 Workout Anatomy

I still remember my first day at the gym. The trainer told me I had to be there three times a week to see results. But even three times a week seemed huge to me back then. "Can I come just twice?" I hesitantly asked.

A lot has changed since then. And I've discovered for myself that three times a week of strength training is just right. Why? Because you don't need more than that to work your muscles. That doesn't mean that you cannot do more, but that's up to you—it's extra credit. You'll soon see for yourself that three times a week is enough to sculpt your body. I know that many popular workout programs suggest exercising five times a week, but seriously, who follows those one month later? Plus, with High Intensity Interval Training, it might be unwise to push your body to 90% of max heart rate more often than three times a week, especially if you're new to exercise.

According to the USA's Department of Health Physical Activity Guidelines for Americans, USDA's Choose My Plate, American Heart Association, and the United Kingdom's National Health Service, it's recommended that adults spread out moderate or vigorous aerobic activity (interval training) over three days a week instead of every day because it helps in muscle recovery, increases the chance of sticking with an exercise plan, and brings the least injury risk. Similarly, weightlifting two days a week instead of every day is preferred for the same reasons.[18] [19] [20] [21]

As explained before, here's my recommendation. Do your 16 minutes of strength and cardiovascular exercise with FB16 three times a week and then follow up with "easy-going" exercise to counter the adverse effects of sitting.

18 U.S. Dept. of Health and Human Services, Physical Activity Guidelines for Americans, 2008. http://www.health.gov/paguidelines/pdf/adultguide.pdf
19 United States Department of Agriculture. ChooseMyPlate. http://www.choosemyplate.gov/physical-activity/amount.html
20 American Heart Association. 2014. http://www.heart.org/HEARTORG/GettingHealthy/PhysicalActivity/FitnessBasics/American-Heart-Association-Recommendations-for-Physical-Activity-in-Adults_UCM_307976_Article.jsp
21 UK National Health Services. 2013. http://www.nhs.uk/Livewell/fitness/Pages/physical-activity-guidelines-for-adults.aspx

Sitting is the new smoking, and if you're like most people, you have a desk job and spend eight or more hours a day sitting. This poses a great risk to your health. It's time to stop it.

Add more movement to your life: gardening, dusting, or walking, it's up to you. What matters is that you spend less time on a chair. Take mini-breaks at work just to stand up and stretch. I've created the Office Exercise and Stretch mobile app (Android and Windows 8) just to help you do that. Small changes can have a big effect on your overall health, vitality, and longevity.

Okay, so by now you know you'll be working out three times a week, and you know that each workout lasts 16 minutes. But what exactly will you be doing each time? Let's dive in.

The four-minute rounds

Every 16-min FB16 workout includes four rounds of exercise, each lasting a total of four minutes. You'll be starting out with round one and two, and you'll then be repeating these two rounds to complete your 16 minutes. During the first round of each workout, I want you to take it easy—this is your warm-up round. Starting from round two, we pick up the pace. In rounds three and four, we go full speed and give it our all. Before you know it, 16 minutes will be up and it'll all be over. Good job!

The FB16 interval training protocols

The most common interval protocols included in FB16 are the 20-10, the 50-10, and the 30-30. In a 20-10 protocol, you'll be doing 20 seconds of intense exercise followed by 10 seconds of rest. Then you'll be moving on to the next exercise for another 20 seconds, followed by another 10 seconds of rest. This will continue until you complete a round of four minutes. Similarly, a 50-10 protocol includes 50 seconds of intense exercise that are followed by 10 seconds of rest.

Now, a 30-30 protocol is a little different. In this protocol, you're quickly alternating between exercises for 3.5 minutes. You then have your 30-second break and complete your four-minute round.

Say you're doing push-ups. You'll do as many as you can for 30 seconds, and then you'll be quickly moving on to the next exercise, say squats. You'll do as many squats as you can for 30 seconds, and then you'll move on to the next exercise. You'll keep switching between exercises for 3 minutes and 30 seconds. And that's when you'll have 30 seconds of rest and complete the round.

Then, there is the combo round, where you play with protocols. In a combo round, you may be doing 30 seconds of one exercise then 20 seconds of another exercise followed by 10 seconds of rest; then you may do another 30 seconds of a third exercise and so on. As long as it adds up to four, you can be creative with how you structure each round.

The complexity with interval training lies in actually measuring time, so that you know exactly when you should be switching exercises. To make things simpler for you, the only two protocols used in the workout plan of this book are the 30-30 and the 20-10. I've also created an interval timer with the workouts already preloaded at http://fitnessreloaded.com/interval-timer/, so that you can simply choose your workout and then let the computer count the time for you!

The protocols might seem short, but if you push yourself enough, then they are just right. So if you're doing 30 seconds of push-ups, don't do slow push-ups (and of course, don't cheat!). Instead, do as many as you can while keeping the right form. Go as fast as you can. Are we doing 20 seconds of high knees? Hop from one leg to the other as fast as you can, bringing your knee as high as you can. This *is* High Intensity Interval Training after all.

Stretching for cooling down

In your fourth round, you'll be going full speed, getting your heart rate quite high. Once done, you'll probably need a few minutes to get your heart rate down to normal and cool down. That's a great opportunity to stretch. I personally prefer to walk around for a minute after I finish working out and then follow up with stretching. Whether you want to put in those two to three minutes to stretching or head to the shower directly is up to you.

Gear Recommendations

What do you really need to do an FB16 workout? Here's the recommended gear.

Must-have: an interval timer

FB16 needs your attention—down to the second. If you don't already have an interval timer to count exercise and rest periods, then no worries. I've built one for you. Go to http://fitnessreloaded.com/interval-timer/ and bookmark this page. Select your workout, or just the protocol you want to follow, and you're good to go!

Shoes or no shoes?

Some workouts are performed with athletic shoes on. Others are done barefoot. What should you do with FB16? I believe there are three issues to consider: your floor type, whether you'll be working on your balance or doing jumps, and safety.

Let's start with what a difference your home's floor type can make. Here's my personal experience. My current home has carpet on the floor. I'm used to working out without shoes because I don't really need them.

So I did that at my parents' house in Greece. I worked out with FB16 on a hard, tile-covered floor. The result? My knees hurt later. The hard surface at my parents' home didn't absorb the energy from the jumping movements of FB16, resulting in mild knee pain—even though I landed softly and followed the right form. Lesson learned. I make sure I always put my athletic shoes on when I'm working out on a hard-surfaced floor.

Another issue to consider is balance. Usually, working out without shoes helps you maintain a better balance. If your FB16 workout has no jumping movements, and especially if it includes balance exercises, then you might find it easier to balance on your bare feet. After all, there's a reason balance-focused workouts like yoga are done barefoot.

Finally, shoes serve to protect your feet from falling objects. Imagine doing a workout with dumbbells and one of your dumbbells falling on your bare foot. Ouch! That's exactly why most gyms only allow working out with athletic shoes on and don't allow admittance if you're wearing sandals or any other shoe. It's a safety concern.

Mat or no mat?

FB16 is heavy on bodyweight exercises, which by default means lots of time on the floor. Whether you use a yoga mat or not is up to you and your floor type. I've found that a mat is absolutely necessary when working out on a hard floor. It's more comfortable to lie on the floor, plus doing burpees, push-ups, tricep dips, or planks becomes easier on your wrists and knees with a mat rather than without one.

Again, on my carpet-covered floor, I don't need a mat. But whenever I work out on a hard floor, I really miss my mat when I don't have it with me.

A chair or other sturdy furniture

Some FB16 workouts are assisted by a chair or another piece of sturdy furniture. We use the chair for balance support, or in the case of exercises like the "chair lunges," to just make lunges exponentially harder and work our muscles more deeply.

Dumbbells

Your own body is your best workout tool, and that's exactly why FB16 is mainly comprised of bodyweight exercises. You literally won't need anything in order to work out other than your own body. But the fact that bodyweight exercises are so effective doesn't mean we shouldn't use weights to further enhance our workouts. Add to those bodyweight exercises dumbbell work, and the results become dramatically better.

Let's be honest—it's hard to have the same level of precision when working your upper body without dumbbells. Dumbbells give your muscle that little extra something, not to mention that weight lifting movements resemble and prepare you for movements you do in your everyday life.

For example, imagine you're holding a baby in your arms. Your baby is a weight that you're lifting. Lifting dumbbells will help prepare you for that. Or imagine you're lifting the grocery bags out of the trunk; you hold everything with one hand while you're closing your trunk with your other hand and then walk to your house. Again, this is you lifting weights. Let's prepare and make everyday life so much easier!

For FB16, I recommend you have two sets of weights: a lighter 2–5 lb. set for shoulder-work, and a heavier 5–10 lb. set for everything else. You'll be alternating between the two when you focus on your upper body.

Cushion

If you're new to the C-position abs, a series of ab exercises you'll find in the abs section, then I recommend you use a cushion to support your low back as you lean to the back. Many people tend to excessively arch their back, which both ruins the form of the exercise and makes them prone to low back pain. Using a cushion right behind your back will help you avoid this mistake so that you develop abs of steel without risking injury.

How FB16 Differs From Other Workouts

FB16 targets your abs and butt while redesigning your whole body. It combines high intensity interval training, isometric exercises, bodyweight exercises, weight lifting, yoga poses, and stretches to sculpt your body and completely change your shape. Each one of the workouts raises your heart rate while driving your muscles to fatigue, forcing them to grow and become stronger.

I created FB16 because I recognized my need for a short, effective and fun workout. Unlike products that are developed by people who don't immediately feel the need for them, FB16 was the result of me scratching my own itch. I needed a workout that was efficient and effective, a workout that could be done anywhere, and a workout that was also fun enough for me to keep doing it more than once or twice. But there was a time when I actually had enough of intense interval training. Here's what happened.

By the time I finished shooting the eight-week video FB16 program, I had been working out with FB16 for four months. I had increased my fitness enough so that I could pull off each FB16 workout in front of the camera while still smiling. But my eight-hour shooting days were packed, as I was also shooting other exercise programs. Let's just say each shooting day had a lot of exercise. I had never exercised so much in my life and sometimes I was questioning whether I could pull it all off—and with a smile on my face. Once shooting was over, I thought, "Finally, no more intense interval training! Time to take a much-needed break."

And so I did. I took a break for a month. I kept exercising five days a week: I was going to the gym; I was brisk walking; I was doing home exercise DVDs; I was just not doing FB16. A month later I felt it was time to get back to it. So I put one of my videos on my computer, and I started exercising. After eight minutes, I was completely exhausted. I was out of breath. My face was red. I wanted to stop and just continue my workout with walking! My fitness level was surprisingly low!

I never expected that dropping FB16 for a month would make my fitness level decline so dramatically, especially since I kept exercising. Right at this instance, I experienced exactly how effective FB16 really is. Even though I was exercising five days a week, just because I had stopped FB16, my fitness level had significantly dropped! My husband, witnessing my exhaustion, found the perfect opportunity to tease me, saying I should release the "FB8" rather than the "FB16"! That was a good laugh for him!

I believe this story shows exactly how different FB16's results are compared to most other exercise programs out there. For your information, I did finish the workout that day. After all it was only another eight minutes, how could I not finish? Now let's get a recap of the FB16 benefits compared to doing other workouts.

Efficient and effective

HIIT helps you get an hour's results in just 16 minutes. You could do the exact same exercises randomly, slowly, or you could do them fast but take long breaks in between. But none of those approaches would lead to muscle overload. They wouldn't help your body get noticeably stronger either. And that's why FB16 is based on the HIIT regimen.

Focus on abs and butt

Yes, FB16 is a total body workout. No body part gets left out. But let's face it; it is biased towards giving you a flat belly and a firm butt. The belly and the butt are the two most common "problem areas," and that's exactly why FB16 focuses on getting those body parts toned and defined. Your abs get stronger while your butt and legs get defined. It's a win.

Attention to posture

FB16 is big on posture. Those slouchy backs and rolled shoulders we acquire by sitting at our desks for eight hours a day? Keeping the right form during each exercise will gradually urge your back to straighten up. The result? Less back pain and a taller, more graceful posture. And yes, you'll even make a better first impression to others because the aura you project when you're slouchy versus when you're standing straight has a very different effect, not just on how you feel but on others too. More on posture later in the book.

Balance work

In FB16, we actively try to improve our balance. We train both our bodies and brains to help us develop the extra precision we need in our movements. It's easy to understand why old people need good balance as this prevents them from falling, but what about younger folks? Well, imagine having better control of your movements. You can pick up a toy from the floor while barely balancing on one leg. You can climb the stairs with more precision. Say you run down the hill and hit a rock that throws your ankle in an awkward angle. Having better balancing skills will help you avoid an ankle injury. Not bad, huh?

Focus on form

When following a fast-paced program, it's easy to get carried away and sacrifice form for speed. That's strictly prohibited in FB16. You get constantly reminded of the right form, whether that is "tucking your pelvis in" or not "letting your shoulders hang." In the FB16 video program I have actually shot additional workout breakdowns that show you exactly how to perform each exercise.

   You don't want to risk injuries by not keeping the right form. Plus, the way you work out is the way you build your body, so keeping the right form will not just help you work the right muscles, it'll also shape your body into a taller you with a straighter and more confident posture.

Fun, with meaningful variety

Unlike other HIIT workouts that preach doing the same few exercises continuously for 90 seconds or more, with every FB16 workout, you'll be doing about 15 exercises. That's 15 exercises that you'll repeat twice in a total of 16 minutes. Let's just say you won't get bored.

   At the same time, you won't feel overwhelmed by too many different exercises either. The workouts have found the sweet spot between too many new exercises and familiar exercises so that you keep your interest up without risking getting overwhelmed.

Fast enough so that you won't feel beaten down

I still remember trying to follow an extremely hard-core workout. The trainer had us do the same difficult move for I don't even know how long. I ended up giving up, sitting on the floor, and feeling like a total failure, embarrassed I couldn't keep up and frustrated that I "had" to keep going.

But in FB16, you won't get this experience. And just when you thought you couldn't take it anymore, time is up and we're jumping into the next exercise. Even if you need to take more frequent breaks, since the exercises go by so fast, you're not in danger of indulging in "pity-parties" for more than a few seconds.

Program design discourages cheating

I've seen too many workout videos and DVDs where even the people in the videos are cheating. Push-ups that don't really go low are a very common sight.

In FB16, it's really hard to do that. You see, you only have 16 minutes. No exercise lasts longer than 30 or 50 seconds at most. It's really hard to wing it, because you know, you don't have a long (unknown) amount of time in front of you, where you have to keep doing the same move again and again. You only have another few seconds! Are you *not* going to give it your best? I cannot guarantee that you will but I know you'll be inclined to work harder compared to other exercise programs. The way the FB16 is built encourages you to push yourself. It's the system working in your favor.

Exact match to your fitness level

The FB16 workouts will keep adjusting to your own fitness level. I designed the program so that you'll keep being challenged no matter how many times you've repeated the same workout. With FB16 you can always do it better. You can go lower on squats. You can go faster on high knees. You can fit in more burpees. You can go from half-pushups to full push-ups. You can switch each exercise with any "Kick It Up" variation. You can always keep pushing harder so that the workouts never end up in the "easy-going" category.

At the same time, if you want to take it easier, or if what you see at first is hard, you can always do a modified version of each exercise. You can avoid going too low on squats. You can go slower on high knees instead of faster. You can adjust FB16 so that it fits your fitness level perfectly.

Perfectly sustainable

Few workout programs can claim sustainability. Most workouts are usually too long to keep up with. Some require you to do them five or six times a week. Yet most people don't have five hours a week to spend on exercise. And most importantly, most people don't even need to spend five days a week doing strength training.

Three days a week are more than enough to sculpt your body. That's not to say you shouldn't exercise more than three times a week. Sure, go ahead, go for walks, attend your yoga class. But as far as reshaping your body is concerned, three times a week and just 16 minutes each time is enough. Now, that's sustainable, isn't it?

Compelling, even irresistible

Even when you're tired, it's just hard to resist working out. Once you do an FB16 workout for the first time, you'll immediately feel how deeply it works. Do it once and you're hooked. Even if you come home tired, you'll know that 25 minutes later you'll have completed your workout and your shower. You'll be smelling great in your clean clothes. That's less than half an hour to get amazing results and finish the shower part that follows every workout! How compelling is that? Many previous students have called FB16 "irresistible" and that's for a good reason.

Frequently Asked Questions

You might already have these questions in mind, or they may come up as you work out with FB16. Here we go.

Should I work out every day?

To me, it's more important that you get your three workouts a week done than when you're actually doing them. I'd prefer you to space them out throughout the week, but I don't mind if you do the workouts on three consecutive days. I don't care if you do two on the same day—even though I wouldn't recommend doing three on the same day unless you're already an experienced exerciser. It's up to you. What really matters is that you get them done—each and every week.

I'm sore, should I exercise?

Yes, soreness should not prevent you from exercising. Just try to do a different workout than the one that made you sore so that you work with different muscles of your body.

I'm not sore. Does this mean the workout was not effective?

Soreness is not an indication of how effective your workout was. Soreness, officially known as Delayed Onset Muscle Soreness (DOMS), occurs when you get microscopic tears in your muscles when training. If you're not sore, but felt the "burn" when you exercised; if you experienced shaking, or you had any other signs of muscle tiredness like feeling too weak to go down the stairs of your house; then you deeply worked those muscles, and luckily didn't tear any muscle fibers.

   Bottom line: You may get sore after doing a fairly simple activity just because it was completely new to you, or you may not get sore after doing a very hard workout—because your body was ready for it!

How should I breathe?

The rule of thumb is inhaling while doing the easier part of the movement and exhaling when doing the harder part of each exercise. For example, with ab work, exhale as you're contracting your abs and inhale as you're releasing to go back to starting position.

I'd advise you not to worry a lot about breathing though. As long as you're not holding your breath, it's hard to go wrong with it because your body is automatically regulating it.

What aesthetic changes should I expect as I keep exercising?

Follow the workout plan presented in this book for four weeks straight, and you'll witness noticeable difference in your energy levels right away. You'll feel stronger and fitter. What used to tire you will now appear much tamer.

Don't expect a magic bullet. FB16 is no magic diet pill that supposedly changes your whole body overnight. Exercise is a lifestyle change. You'll see more and more results as you keep doing those workouts. You'll be surprised by the changes and by the extent to which your body changes shape. I've had people lose 20 pounds in eight weeks just from exercising three times a week with FB16. But the weight is just one change; witnessing your legs becoming thinner, your butt getting a lift, your love handles shrinking, and your middle becoming slimmer is an amazing experience. And it's all about to start happening now.

Here's what Joseph Pilates said about pilates: "After 10 sessions you will feel the difference. After 20 sessions you will see the difference. After 30 sessions others will notice the difference!" Now considering FB16 is really fast in producing results, how does this quote translate for you? Here's what I've seen from FB16 students so far:

- Week Two - Notice a big difference in the way you feel and a slightly noticeable difference in the way you look—mostly the type of changes that other people can't notice yet but you can!
- Week Four - Notice real differences in your body. Your closest friends or partner might notice too.
- Week Six - More people start spotting the difference as well! Compliments are coming!

- Week Eight and beyond - The longer you stick to FB16 the more you'll be reshaping your body. Keep working out and your body will be completely resculpted. Your physique will completely change! Your legs will look better when you wear skirts or shorts, your arms will look different when you wear sleeveless tops, and every bit of your body will change.

Will my body type change?

No. For example, I have a Mediterranean body type with naturally big hips and thighs. No matter what I do or what I eat, I can never look like Cameron Diaz, who has a totally different body type. No matter what she does, she can also never get the natural curves my body gives me. She cannot look like me. These are natural limitations.

But what we can both do is look as best as we can and show off the best of our body type. Get this? Beauty comes in all shapes and sizes. So if you have a pear-shaped body with natural curves, then you can either look like a delicious, toned pear or like a saggy, disproportionate pear. The same is true if you have an apple-shaped body. You can look amazing or not-so-amazing. Nothing can change your body type or bone structure, but exercise is the ticket to looking your personal best!

Are there any dietary recommendations?

I don't want to do a B job on diet by throwing some recipes in this book and pretending I covered an issue as complicated and hotly debated as diet. That's why I chose to keep *Flat Belly Firm Butt in 16 Minutes* strictly to exercise. This is not a weight loss manual; it's a results-focused workout plan.

I do have a diet-related recommendation though. Are you drinking enough water? Mayo Clinic suggests 2.2 liters (9 cups) for women and 3 liters (13 cups) for men. If not, then it's time to make drinking more water a habit. (Don't know how to create healthy habits? Search for "Maria Brilaki" on Amazon to check out my best-selling book that details exactly this topic.) Add 1.5 to 2.5 cups of water for the days when you're exercising.

Is there anything else I should know before I get started?
Familiarize yourself with the exercises first. Here's why. FB16 is time sensitive. You do one exercise after the other and have absolutely zero time to open this book and try to understand exactly what you need to do, where your hand should be placed, or exactly what movement you're doing with your leg.

In the eight-week exercise program, I've included separate "breakdowns" for each workout so that you know exactly how to perform each move before the workout starts. Once you perform these exercises a few times, you'll know them so well that you'll cruise from one exercise to the other without needing to first consult the book (or the breakdown if you're doing the video program).

Got more questions? Contact me and my team at fitnessreloaded.com/contact.

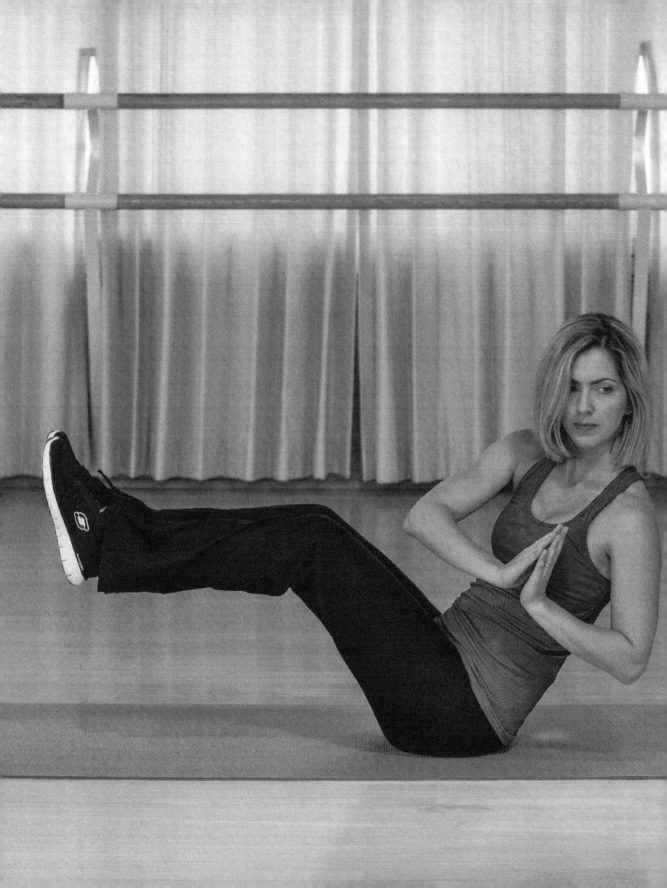

THE FB16 MIND

We are accustomed to thinking that to succeed, we need to take action. That's true, but it's not the whole truth. In reality, taking action alone is not enough. Taking action with the wrong mindset can actually be both a huge struggle and completely counterproductive—not just in fitness but in anything in life. But when we take action with the right mindset in place, that's when we achieve the results we want in the fastest and most enjoyable way possible.

At Fitness Reloaded, we do things differently. We openly recognize that success in any endeavor—including fitness—doesn't just come from taking physical action; the right mindset is a necessary component to success. And that's why in this section, I'll give you guidelines on how to build the right mindset to perfectly complement the FB16 workout program.

But before I get to the mental guidelines, let's first examine what happens in life when you don't take care of how you think:

A 45-year-old lady who wants to lose weight
She gets on a weight-loss program, and she pushes herself hard. In six months she has lost tens of pounds and is very happy with her weight loss. However, a year later she has gained all the weight back plus some more. She thinks, "I tortured myself, I struggled, I lost it, and now it is back! What am I doing wrong?"

A 25-year-old guy who wants to find love
He doesn't like being single, and he wants to find love, but he is so desperate about it that the ladies know. If you sound desperate and needy, no lady is going to go on a date with you. So even though he applies a lot of effort to go talk to girls, finds the courage to do it, and says all the "right" things, he keeps getting rejected because he sounds too needy. So he thinks, "I am trying hard. I get no results. What am I doing wrong?"

A 35-year-old woman who wants to start her own business

She is not too happy with her job and has a dream of doing her own business on the side. But she doesn't really know how to do it, and it just seems so complex and overwhelming that she can't seem to get started. She has been thinking about it for the last five years but just doesn't take any action. She says, "Yeah, now is not the right time…maybe later." She is still stuck in her job. Still no action. Still no progress. She's stuck asking herself, "what am I doing wrong?"

Now let me ask you: What do you think all these three people have in common? I know you're suspecting "wrong mindset" as an answer, but let's dig into this deeper. I'll give you a second to think about this. Okay, three seconds. One, two, three… Well, let me tell you the answer.

All of them tortured themselves. The lady who wanted to lose weight tortured herself on her diet. She tried to force the outcome. The same is true with our second example. This guy wanted to get dates but was trying too hard. That is why he came across as needy and desperate and no girl wanted to go out with him. As for the lady who wanted to start her own business, she made it so overwhelming and big that of course she was going to cringe when even thinking about it.

Dreams are supposed to make us happy about the possibilities and opportunities that are out there, but the way many of us think about them not only makes us unhappy, but also makes us overwhelmed about what to do first, frustrated that we're not there already, or paralyzed to even start.

None of the three people in the above examples have success-optimized mindsets. If you have a mindset like theirs, then your dreams and goals are at risk:

- You will never get started.
- You will waste your time doing the wrong things, putting so much effort in but getting little in return.

That's exactly why the lady who really pushed herself got results. But then again, she also lost everything because her mindset was not up-to-speed. If she was excited about going on this weight loss program and said, "Yes, I am going to love what is going to happen in the next six months. I can't wait!" her story would have had a whole different ending. But she wasn't. Instead, she had to force herself to lose weight. She put in too much effort, but ended up with little results.

But how could she like losing weight, you may ask. How could she like something that didn't feel good? Well, that's what we'll be discussing in this section of the book.

Same Action, Different Results

Take two people, Tom and Jerry (any similarities to a popular cartoon are completely accidental). They are two identical men. They both want to lose weight, and get on the same weight loss plan. They both start a daily, 30-minute walking practice in addition to their eating diet. What they do differently, though, is the way they think. They think differently about everything they do to lose weight, including their walking practice.

When Tom goes out for a walk, he's doing it because he "has to." Sometimes he even wonders why he gets into this trouble. After all, 30 minutes of walking is not going to be more than 150 calories. So why bother for the equivalent of one and a half bananas?

When Jerry goes out for a walk, he's excited he'll be putting a checkmark on his daily walking practice. Sure, 150 calories is not going to make or break his weight loss success, but it will help. Plus, he read once that people who exercise when on a diet tend to keep the weight off more than those who only diet. So yes, it's a hassle to go out and walk sometimes; no, it's not going to give tremendous instant benefits, but it is "one more brick" on the "thinner Jerry" wall.

Now here are my questions to you:
- Who is happier while losing weight, Tom or Jerry?
- Who has a higher chance of actually following through with the weight loss plan and getting results, Tom or Jerry?
- Who is more likely to do more (e.g., walk more) with time, Tom or Jerry?
- Who has higher chances of keeping the weight off after the diet is over, Tom or Jerry?
- Whose way of thinking helps him become unstoppable and get anything he wants, Tom's or Jerry's?

Mindset is a game changer. In Tom's case, even if he has his hands on the best diet and exercise plan in the whole world, he's still at risk of spoiling it all because of the way he thinks.

Jerry, on the other hand, is the type of person who will get results, even if his plan is not optimal. Why? Because he has a winner mindset. He accepts limitations without feeling discouraged by them. He's realistic and optimistic at the same time. He doesn't look for a magic bullet that will immediately change everything. He's doing what he can, even if it's only another brick. He doesn't care how small or big the action is—as long as it builds his wall, he's happy to take one more step ahead.

Now it might be easy to see that Jerry is more likely to succeed than Tom when it's all written down like that and in plain sight. It's just easy to understand that Jerry and Tom will get completely different results, even though in theory, right now, they are following the exact same action plan.

But what about us? What if we happen to be more like Tom than Jerry? How can we switch the way we think to become more like Jerry? I first realized how important mindset was years ago when I got started with mindfulness. Since then, I cannot help but notice the big correlation between my Tom-like and Jerry-like thoughts and my success—or lack thereof.

- Tom-like thoughts would make me feel that I couldn't really change the future, so why bother anyway? So I would take less action. And yes, less action meant fewer results.
- Jerry-like thoughts would make me feel that I could change the future, even though this change wouldn't be instant. I knew I had power to do anything I wanted in my hands, and I told myself I'd better use it! And I did! And that's how results came!

Obviously, this mindset does not just affect health. It affects everything: Getting to the next level career-wise, writing a book, getting better relationships, etc. In order to teach myself to be more like Jerry and less like Tom, I started experimenting. After lots of trial and error and after reading everything I could on mindset, I found techniques that worked consistently. The Christmas Principle is one of the best.

The Christmas Principle

So what is the Christmas Principle? Feeling excitement instead of fear, feeling eagerness instead of overwhelm, or feeling optimism instead of pessimism. Thinking of your goal or dream and feeling "yes" or "wow" rather than "I don't know," "impossible," "no way," "but what if," "how do I know that," etc.

You can only have one feeling state at a time. For example, you cannot be super-excited but feel doubtful too. If you have intense positive feelings, by default you cannot at the same time feel self-doubt, fear, worry, and the other members of the negativity gang. This optimistic mindset is your ticket to achieving any goal quickly. No, I'm not telling you to wear rose-colored glasses. After all, Jerry did not wear any. I would argue that his view of reality was more accurate than Tom's; Tom would criticize everything and distort anything positive in an effort to make it seem meaningless, while Jerry would see the true value of his actions. Jerry was more of a realist than Tom.

The Christmas Principle is the difference between exercising because you hate your body and your own skin versus exercising because you want to look and feel amazing. It's the difference between dieting and looking forward to fitting in your old jeans versus dieting because you absolutely can no longer stand the way you look. It's like spotting a very fit person and being inspired by their example versus getting depressed because seeing this person only reminds you how far away you are from this dream.

It is like sitting in a very pretty car. You've always wanted this car, but experiencing this car doesn't make you excited. Instead, it reminds you of how crappy your current car is. Instead of enjoying the moment, and feeling energized by this experience, you feel bad. The nice car dream makes you feel really bad about yourself and your current situation. You get bogged down. This is not a good place to be if you care about actually having (and not just dreaming about) a better car!

Okay, so you get the principle. But why do I call it the "Christmas" Principle? Because each one of us got it right when we were little. I mean, we still do get it right quite often, but when we were little, we were pros at it.

Let me freshen up your memory. When you were a kid and you were expecting your Christmas presents, did this idea of a Christmas present make you feel anxious or worried? Did it make you think, "Oh crap, it is not Christmas Day today"? Or did it make you feel eager and excited about what this present would be? I think you were happy. I think you loved dreaming about the arrival of Christmas. You loved fantasizing how you would run to the Christmas tree, open your present, see what was inside, and then spend the day playing with your toys.

You were actually very eager and excited about Christmas even months before December. In November, you were not beating yourself up because it was not Christmas Day yet. You were really looking forward to Christmas, but your eagerness did not make you stress about the date not yet being December 25. You see, when you were a kid, you had the right mindset—the winning one.

But you might say, "Of course I'd get a present. There was no uncertainty in that." Give me a break. You believed in Santa Claus! You just believed. If you doubted Santa Claus would come, then believe me, you wouldn't have felt so excited about Christmas. You might have even been worried—would you really get a present? What if all kids got one except for you? Oh, you could have been worried, but again, if you were like most kids, you probably were not worried at all! You expected the best! And that's how you could be happy about Christmas even before Christmas!

Whenever I ponder about the Christmas Principle, I cannot avoid thinking that we humans are so weird. All we want is happiness—a better body, house, or relationship are only means to more happiness. Yet even though happiness is the ultimate goal, we choose a goal-setting process that tortures us. We beat ourselves up when we don't progress as much as we want. We feel anxious. We feel worried. We whip ourselves to work and try harder to go for our dream. In the end, even though we want what we want because we think it will make us happier, we think it is okay to make ourselves feel bad in the present moment to get the elusive happiness later. And once we achieve the goal, we get happy for a little while, until we set the next goal and go back to being stressed and worried and unhappy. Aren't we humans such smarty pants?

Now, of course, as shown in the Tom and Jerry example, worrying and doubting is a recipe for few—or no—results. But apart from the results, isn't it weird that even though what we want is happiness, we're willing to beat ourselves up to get it?

Now, if you apply the Christmas Principle and you feel excited and optimistic about what's coming rather than fearful or doubtful, then you're on the fastest lane to success. First, you will actually get started. You will not procrastinate because you don't know where to start or because it seems too big. You will take action. And action done with the right mindset brings results!

Second, you will naturally choose the right things to do. You will make good decisions—decisions that propel you forward and don't keep you trapped doing meaningless things. Fear or doubt encourage you to play small, so most decisions made from that place of lack are rarely (if ever) the optimal ones. Just compare the decisions you make when you're optimistic (let's find a way to make it happen!) versus the decisions you make when you're pessimistic (why try anyway?). Enough said.

So now let's cover the next topic: If your fitness goal doesn't make you feel excited but instead fills you with fear, doubt, or overwhelm, then what do you do?

Three Scripts to Reprogram Your Mind

How do you feel better about your fitness goal if your goal does not exactly fill you with joy right now? How do you live the Christmas Principle no matter what? Well, below are the three most common negative scripts that come up when we exercise and exactly how to overwrite them.

"I hate where I'm at right now."
Scripts that emphasize how bad our current situation is are so common. They make us feel powerless and overwhelmed. They bring stagnation because any attempt to change the situation seems futile. Replace this with: "The present is the result of the past. What I do today will shape what I get tomorrow."

Think about it. Isn't it true that how your body currently looks or how much endurance you currently have is a result of the past? Your present situation is only a reflection of what you did the day before, the month before, etc. Your present situation has nothing to do with who you really are now and what you can achieve today!

This is like looking at the night sky. The stars you see? They are not really there. This is only a reflection of the past. Since it takes years for the light to reach the earth, what you see in the night sky is how the stars looked like many years ago. Some of those stars may be bigger. Others may have even died. But you can't see that, can you? Because you only see the past.

It is the same with your body and current fitness level. This is only a result of the past and has absolutely no relation to who you are right now.

"How do I know things will be different this time?"
Ugh, self-doubt. Why go through the trouble to make our dreams come true when there's no guarantee? It's better not to try in the first place.

Self-doubt is so smart! She seems reasonable, even protective, but in reality, she's stabbing us in the back, keeping our most meaningful dreams away from us. Let's change this: "What happened before is irrelevant. The future is in my hands."

You're not the same person as you were before. You now know more. You have more experience. You have more clarity on what you want and what works for you. Even if you don't immediately succeed, you'll still gain more experience and clarity to do it better next time. There's no loss really. You're walking on a staircase where every step leads to better and better clarity. You're not the same person you were ten steps ago. Things looked different back then. The view was different. Because of your experience, you now have the best perspective you've ever had in your whole life, and it's up to you to put it to good use.

"But I have to face reality!"
You feel like you have to see things "as they are." You might think you're too fat, or too broke, or too something. And that's how things are—you cannot deny that!

And it might be true. Your BMI reflects obesity, and your bank account is on the verge of suicide. But focusing upon the problem only makes you feel powerless, overwhelmed, or depressed. None of those feelings actually help you lower your BMI or get money in your account. They mostly push you to never try to change the situation, as reality seems too strong to change. But is it really? Or is this another treacherous way of thinking? Replace this with: "Yes, things are not perfect right now, but reality is only temporary. Life is shifting all the time."

Think about it. Life is shifting whether you want it to or not. You once were a baby, you grew up, maybe went to college, maybe had kids. The only constant is change. Your life keeps changing. And so will you. Nothing is too permanent; instead, everything is shifting, regardless of whether you see it or not. Even if things are not perfect right now, you can change that. You can help guide the changes that are currently happening in your life so that your life changes the way you want it to.

Whenever you find yourself thinking one of those three scenarios, refer to this page and read the antidote script. The more you do it, the more you will reprogram your mind so that you make this new way of thinking a habit! Make applying the Christmas Principle a habit, and you'll be developing a winner's mindset that gets you the results you want—and fast!

Remove the Weeds

And just in case the previous scripts were not enough, I'm going to give you even more specific instructions to really make sure that the wrong mindset will not hold you back from success.

Picture your mind like a garden: If the weeds take over, there will be no space for flowers or nutritious vegetables. Self-judgmental thoughts and self-doubt both belong in the weeds category, and they are prohibited in FB16. Yes, you read that right. Prohibited. Here's a list of the most common FB16-related weeds:

- How few repetitions we do.
- Beating ourselves up for not going low on squats.
- Whether we should have already progressed further.
- How bad our balance is.
- How many breaks we take.
- Why we hadn't started exercising years ago.
- Whether we'll ever get the results we want.
- Whether we look silly doing all this stuff or how our bodies look when we exercise—whether we seem fat or our butt looks bad.
- We've never really liked exercise—who are we kidding?

Bad, bad weeds. They only take your focus away from the present moment. And the present moment is beautiful. It's you practicing your workout, doing something that is good for you and your body. Don't let any other thought tell you otherwise! Take your shovel:

- If you only manage to do three repetitions, pat yourself on the back for giving it your best, and enjoy your rest!
- If you cannot go low on squats, be happy because those muscles get stronger with every workout!
- If you think you should have progressed further, then know that your body is doing exactly what you need and at the right time. You currently have more than a trillion different cells managing your very existence,

which results in you breathing and speaking and moving and thinking. Their cooperation is perfect, and that's why you're still alive. You think they can't handle you working out or that you know better than them? Just imagine getting one trillion people and making them collaborate perfectly. *Right.*

- If you lose your balance, pat yourself on the back for trying, and then try again. You wouldn't yell at a one-year-old for not walking perfectly already, would you? Why should you be good at this when you've never practiced it before?

- When your body asks for breaks, take them. Again, don't try to be the manager on what your body should or shouldn't do. Your cells know better than you what you need, so you better follow their guidance. It's a break then! Ahhh…

- So you didn't exercise before, but you're doing it now! It's awesome that you're into exercise. These good feelings will help you keep this up. Remember this thought if you ever, ever consider quitting. Oh, and if you worry about the damage done to your body already because you didn't exercise before, then just remember that even the smokers' lungs remove the dirt when smokers stop smoking. Your body knows what to do. Your job is to keep it up!

- Worrying about the timing of results? Keep exercising and you'll see for yourself exactly when you'll get the results you want.

- Are you really silly? Who's the judge? Kids look silly too, but we call them funny. I think it's funny when I lose my balance. Thinking you look silly— or fat—usually comes from hating something about your body. Please remind yourself that reality is only temporary. Your life is always changing. No one should have the power to prevent you from doing something good for you, not even your own thoughts. Take your power back, and do what you have to do.

- So you've never really liked exercise, but you never did FB16 before, right? This is your very first time trying this. Approach it with fresh eyes and an open heart.

Okay, so you're now weed-free. But beware, weeds will come up again. Just like in any garden, where you need to regularly clean up the weeds, it is similar with your mind. Have your shovel somewhere handy because you'll be using it again soon!

A weed-free environment will help you be consistent with FB16. Consistency will give you the results you want. Seeing those results will make you happy and encourage you to keep exercising. As you keep it up, you'll see more results, which will also make you happy and encourage you to keep going, bringing you even more results. You see where I'm going with this here? That's the wheel of unstoppability. Once you get on it, nothing can bring you down.

Except for weeds. So have your shovel somewhere handy, and bookmark this chapter for future reference.

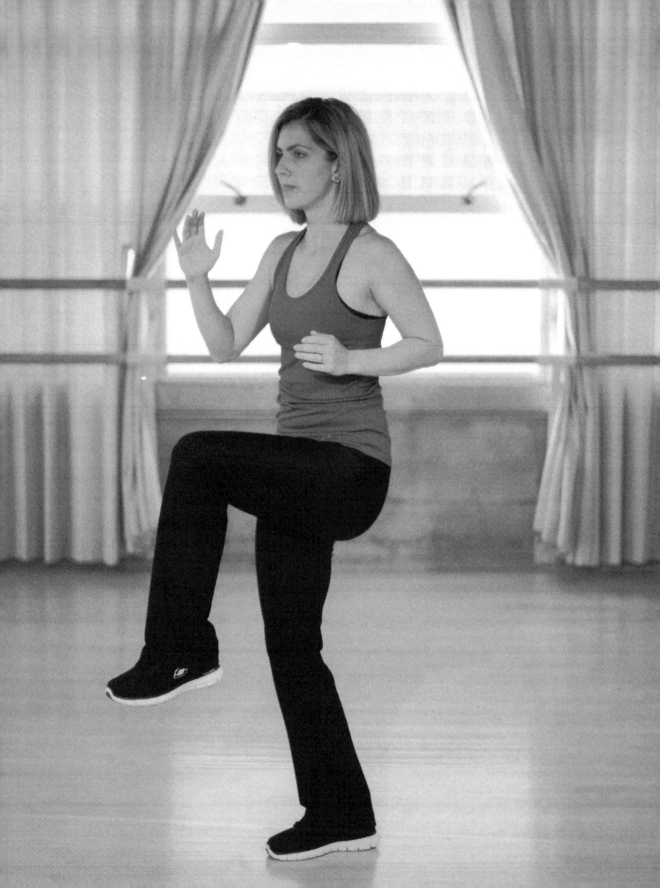

THE FB16 BODY

You worked your mind, now let's work your body. We're now ready to cover the amazing exercises that earned their way into the FB16 program. In this section, I'll show you step-by-step instructions on how to preform each move. Moves are broken down into different sections:

- Home Cardio Exercises
- Abs Exercises
- Legs & Butt Exercises
- Upper Body Exercises
- Balance Exercises
- Queen Burpees
- Cool Down

It was hard to categorize exercises, as some of them fit multiple categories. High knees, for example, is an amazing cardio exercise that also happens to work your core quite deeply. Push-ups are mostly known for their upper-body miracles, but in reality, they are an amazing ab exercise as well. Most exercises in the Balance section would be a great fit for the Legs & Butt section. Burpees get their own section because they are the most amazing multi-muscle moves you could ever do.

I also made sure to include both easier and harder variations of each exercise. This way, it's easy for you to make a workout harder or easier and fine-tune it to your own fitness level. Now, before we get acquainted with each move, let's first cover the basics.

THE POSTURE

With FB16, I want you to stand up for yourself. Literally. Let's admit it: Most of us slouch the whole day with rounded backs and rounded shoulders. Many of us experience back pain as a result. But that's just one effect of poor posture. Poor posture also:

- Makes us shorter. A slouchy posture costs you in inches. It is not a coincidence that people gain one to two inches in height after starting exercise programs that emphasize having a straight posture (think yoga).
- It emphasizes your belly fat. When you stand straight, the belly fat stretches out and appears smaller. When you slouch, the belly fat protrudes more and appears bigger. Note in my posture pictures in this chapter how different my belly looks. Then go in front of a mirror and see this effect for yourself.

If you're like most people, you might have never thought about straightening your posture as a valid way to look thinner. Talk about getting results without diet or exercise! Most of us connect diet and exercise with looking better and rarely if ever consider the shape of our backs and how it affects our presence.

But a good posture is not just about looks and back pain. A straight posture is also about confidence. Yes, confidence. Your posture affects the way you feel. Standing tall affects our biochemistry, increasing testosterone and decreasing cortisol (the infamous stress hormone). Just like smiling—even when you're faking it—makes you happier, a straighter posture makes you feel more powerful, less stressed, and, yes, unstoppable.

And it's not just that you feel better. It's also that others perceive you more favorably. No, I'm not making things up. Harvard Professor Amy Cuddy[22] has studied this subject extensively, and these are her findings. A good posture helps you make a better first impression, and your chances of getting that job after the interview just go up!

But here's another reason we pay attention to your posture in FB16. The way you work out is the way you build your body. If you're working out with a slouchy posture, then you're actually reinforcing it. Let me explain.

Our muscles adapt to our slouchy posture, creating what is known as "muscle imbalances." Some muscles become stiffer because of it, while other muscles become lengthened and weaker. You see, muscles can only do two things: lengthen or shorten. Take your biceps for example—the muscles in the front of your upper arm. When they shorten (or contract), you lift your lower arm up! That's when those guns show up. When they lengthen, your forearm goes down.

At the same time, the muscles opposite your biceps—your triceps (or the muscles at the back of your upper arm)—are responsible for the opposite movement. So when you want to extend your arm, your triceps shorten, pulling that forearm back; when you want to lift that forearm up, your triceps relax (or lengthen) while your biceps contract.

So when you're holding a baby in your arms, your biceps are shortened, while your triceps are lengthened. Now imagine what would happen if you held a baby for eight or ten hours a day, for years. Your muscles would adapt. Your biceps would become shorter, while your triceps would lengthen—permanently.

Now let's translate this baby-carrying example into posture. When you slouch, your upper back muscles lengthen. Your gluteal muscles and hamstrings weaken. We don't want to reinforce those imbalances in FB16. We want the opposite. So here are two important keys to keep in mind as you're exercising:

22 TedTalks: Your body language shapes who you are. TEDGlobal 2012. http://www.ted.com/talks/amy_cuddy_your_body_language_shapes_who_you_are?language=en

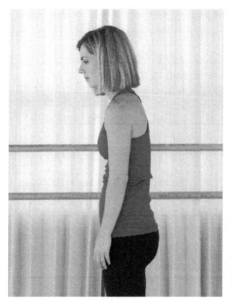 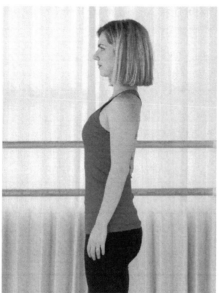

slouchy posture   right posture

First, roll your shoulders back and contract your back muscles to straighten up while you stop curving your upper back.

Second, contract your abs and your butt so that you tuck your pelvis in and reduce the "anterior pelvic tilt." The "anterior pelvic tilt" happens when your gluteal muscles are weakened, and your pelvis has the tendency to "fall forward", creating a bigger curve at your lower back. This curve makes you prone to both lower back pain and injuries. The best way to avoid this is to tuck your pelvis in. You'll have the tendency to forget about this as you're exercising, but with time, it'll become second nature. For example, here's what a wrong and a right squat look like. I'm obviously emphasizing the wrong posture so that the effect is visible.

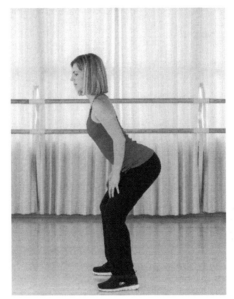

butt is sticking out

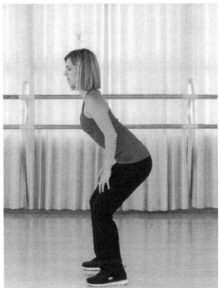

butt is tucked in

In the eight-week FB16 workout program, I'm mentioning it in almost every workout: do not stick your butt out. Even if you think you're not sticking it out, you might be doing it. So contract your abs and your butt, and you should be good to go.

HOME CARDIO
EXERCISES

Cardio. You know…the type of exercise that gets your heart rate up. Well, that's exactly what you'll be doing with the exercises of this section. Enjoy!

WARM-UP **CARDIO**

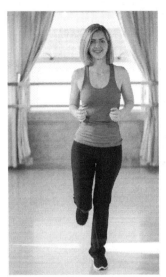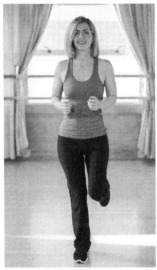

JOG

Jog in place, without actually going somewhere.

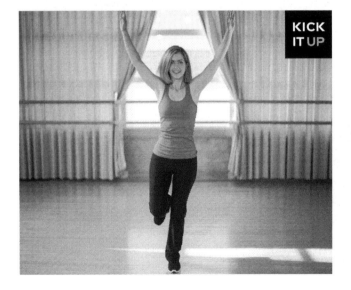

KICK IT UP

JOG
WITH ARM ROLLS

Now let's add arm rolls while jogging in place.

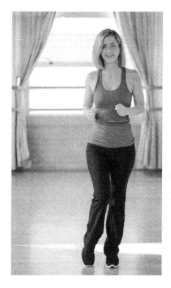
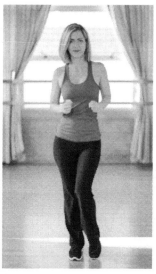

BOXER SHUFFLE

Transfer your weight from one leg to the other as if you were a boxer.

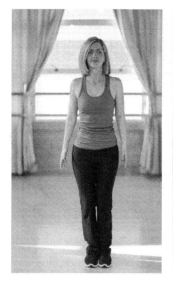
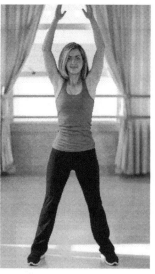

JUMPING JACKS

Start with feet next to each other and arms hanging freely on your sides. Your back should be straight. Jump while you open your legs to more than hip width apart. As you open your legs, you rotate your arms up, bringing your hands together above your head.

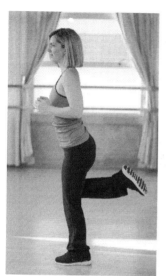 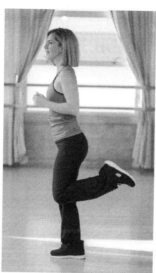

BUTT KICKS

Stand straight with your arms to your sides. Bend one knee, and raise one heel high enough to almost touch your seat. With a slight jump, bring your heel down while you bring the other heel up. Keep alternating.

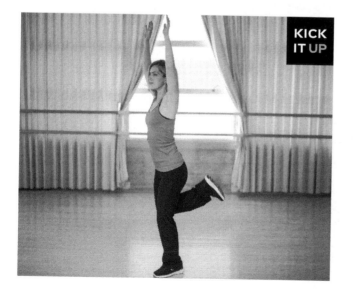

KICK IT UP

BUTT KICKS
WITH ARMS UP

Do butt kicks just like before, but instead of having your arms next to your sides, extend them up above your head.

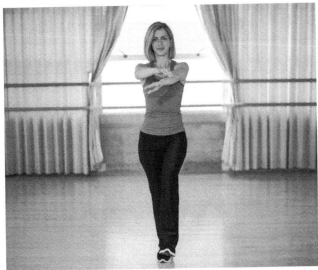

ARMS AND KICKS

Stand straight with your arms extended in front of you. Kick to the front with one leg while slightly crossing your hands. Then kick with your other foot while doing one more crossing movement. Keep it up!

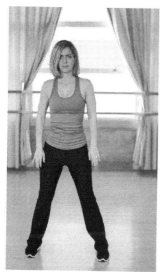
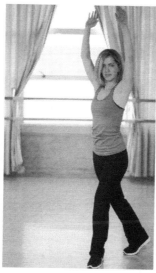
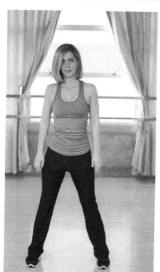
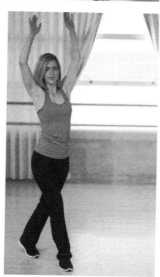

TWIST LUNGE

This is a dance-like movement. Stand straight with your feet more than hip width apart. With your left leg, step to the side and back, placing your foot behind your right leg. Then step back to the center. With your right leg, step behind your left leg. Come back to the center.

To make this exercise harder, we're also adding an arm movement. Your arms are down when you're at the center. You lift them up when you step to the side.

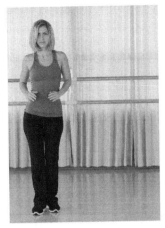
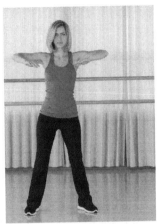

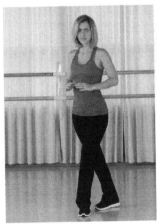
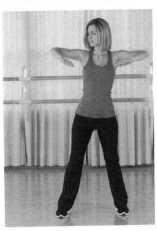

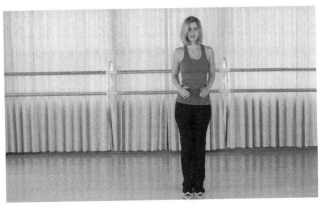

SIDE STEPS

Stand straight with your feet together and your elbows on your sides, bent on a 90-degree angle. Then, step to the right, opening your legs more than hip width apart, while you lift your arms horizontally on shoulder level. Then with your left foot step to the right, placing your left foot behind your right one and at the same time lowering your elbows down.

With your right foot step to the right while you bring your elbows back up on shoulder level. Then bring your feet together and your elbows down to return to starting position. Repeat the movement going to the left side this time. Keep alternating until the time is up.

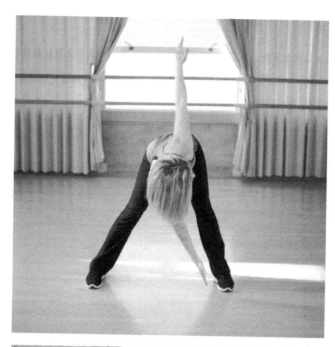

CROSS TOE
TOUCHES

Stand straight with your feet
more than hip width apart. Keep
your back straight. Now bend
from the hip level while keeping
your back straight and extending your arms to the sides.

   Once you form a 90-degree
angle, twist your torso so that
one hand almost reaches the
opposite foot and you push the
other arm up and to the back.
Then twist again so that your
other hand reaches your other
foot.

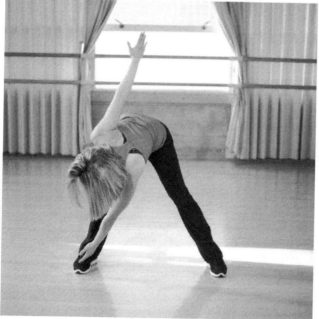

STRENGTHENING CARDIO

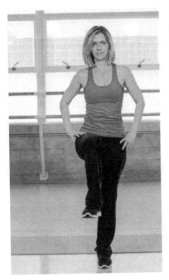
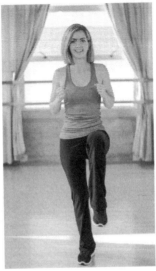
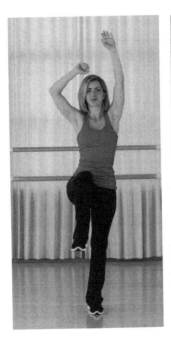
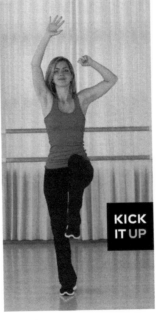

KICK
IT UP

HIGH KNEES

Stand with your feet together. Contract your abs, and lift one knee up until it becomes level with your waist. Then put your foot down and raise the other knee up with a small hopping movement. Repeat. Your back should remain straight at all times; don't slouch, and do not stick your butt out.

Now, how high are high knees really? Here's a simple check to see whether you're winging it or not. Get your arms next to your body, and bend your elbows at a 90 degree angle. Lift your knee up. Does it touch your hand? If not, then you're not lifting your knee high enough.

KNEES AND ARMS

With each leg lift, also raise your arms high as if you're trying to grab something that's high above your head.

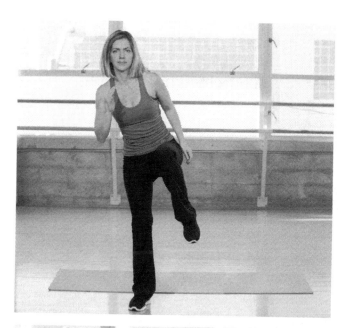

ALTERNATING
JUMPS

With your legs a bit more than hip width apart, lift one leg while you lean towards the opposite side. Then lift the other leg up while you lean towards the other side.

This exercise gets harder as soon as you start jumping from one leg to the other.

As you perform the movement, make sure your butt is tucked in. Do not stick your butt out, but tuck your pelvis in instead.

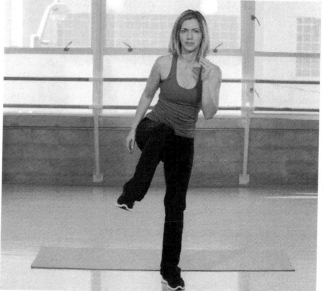

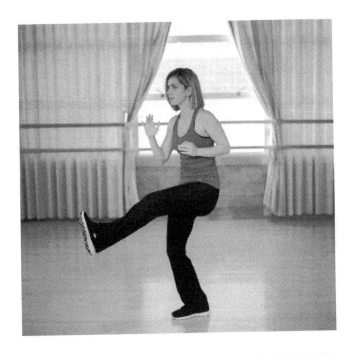

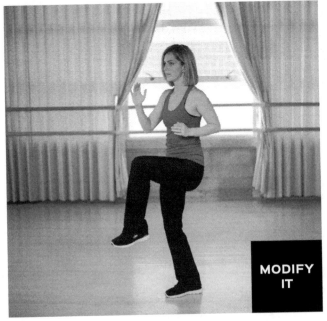

MODIFY
IT

SWITCH KICKS

Stand straight with your knees slightly bent and your fists in front of your face, as if you're protecting yourself in a boxing match. Now stand on one leg while you kick with the other leg. Bring your leg as high as you can. The higher you kick, the harder this exercise becomes. Then bring this leg down while you're kicking up with your other leg.

As you kick, I want you to engage your abs so you really lift your leg up. As you engage your core, your body shape will change a bit, creating a slight curve. Take it up to the next level by picking up the pace and jumping with every kick while switching kicks really fast. Great cardio exercise, right?

HALF SWITCH KICKS

Instead of a full kick, perform a half kick.

RAINBOW

Let's go back to being a five-year-old! In rainbow, you are painting an imaginary rainbow with your fingers. So here's how it works: Start from one side of the "rainbow," bend both legs, touch the floor with your outer hand, then stand up and take one step to the other side of the "rainbow" while both of your arms are extended high above your head. Then again bend your knees and touch the floor with your other arm.

Awesome, now paint another rainbow as you return to starting position. As you perform this movement, your arms paint an imaginary rainbow around your body and come full circle, with one hand touching the floor at the start of the rainbow in the exercise's beginning and your other hand touching the floor at the end of the rainbow at the end of the exercise.

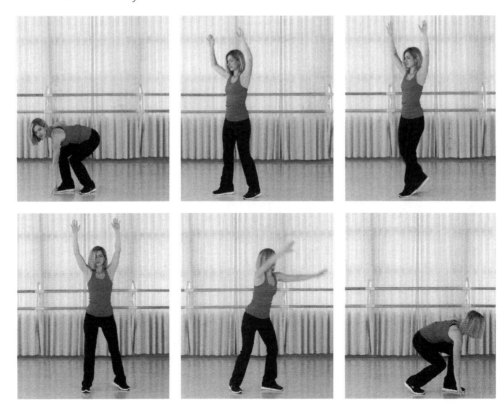

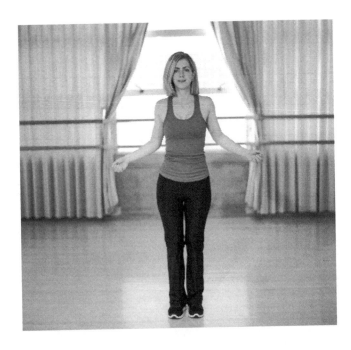

JUMP ROPE

Let's go back to being seven! With both feet together, use an imaginary (or an actual) rope, and jump up with both feet as if you're jumping over it.

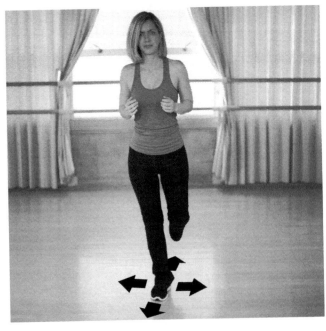

CROSS HOPS

Stand straight with your feet together. Bend one leg at knee level, lifting your heel up, while balancing on one leg only. Now start jumping on one leg, performing a cross on the floor: front, right, back, left. Then repeat for your other leg.

DECK SQUAT JUMPS

I recommend you use a mat for this exercise as you will need a soft place to lie on. Start off with your feet together and your arms being extended. Now squat down, sit back on the floor, and roll on your back with your arms and legs extended. Bring your knees to your chest, and try to get your feet to almost touch the mat. Without using your hands, roll forward until your feet touch the floor, and jump up as high as you can. Repeat the movement.

Make sure you don't put too much pressure on your neck as you slide on your back with your legs on top of you. Practice this movement slowly until you can do it in a controlled manner that doesn't put your neck at risk.

Make it easier by removing the jumping, and instead of keeping your legs extended when you roll on the mat, keep them bent.

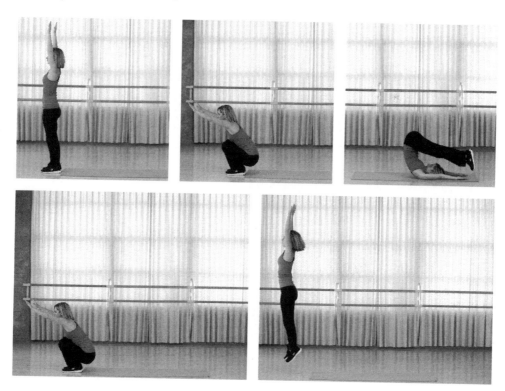

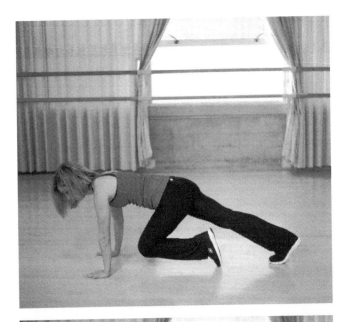

MOUNTAIN
CLIMBERS

Get down into a plank position (see the abs section for details on the plank). Now bend one knee, bringing one leg to the front without actually placing your foot on the floor. Now jump while you alternate legs.

To make it easier, instead of jumping, slow the pace. Just bring one leg to the front then step back without jumping. Repeat.

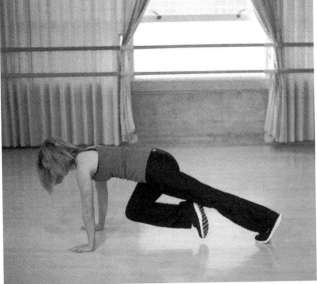

ABS EXERCISES

It sounds like cliché, but I do like the "abs of steel" expression. Just after finishing the shooting of the FB16 eight-week exercise program, I stood next to my husband, who was sitting on a chair. He tried to hug me, and rest his head on my belly. He ended up "hurting" his head on my belly because it was way too firm! Let's just say I had a good laugh!
   Here are the exercises I did to get those abs.

THE **PLANK SERIES**

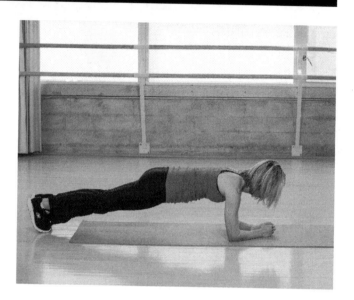

ELBOW PLANK

This is the base exercise for all the plank series. You may also hear it called the "forearm plank." Lay stomach down on the floor with your feet together. Place your elbows under your shoulders, and lift your body up into a straight plank.

Do not push your pelvis up, and do not let your hips sink down. Contract your abs, and hold this position for as long as you can.

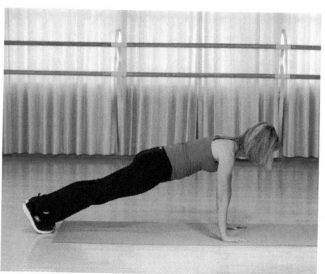

REGULAR PLANK

This is similar to the elbow plank, only harder. Lay stomach down on the floor with your feet together. Place your hands under your shoulders, and lift your body up into a plank. Keep it straight.

Do not push your pelvis up, and do not let your hips sink down. Contract your abs, and hold this position for as long as you can.

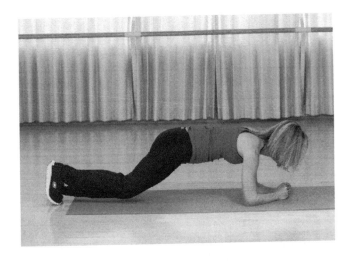

ELBOW PLANK
BEND & STRAIGHTEN

Get into an elbow plank position. Now bend your knees without touching the floor. Then quickly straighten your legs. Repeat.

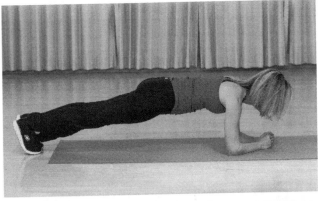

ELBOW PLANK
WITH HIP TWISTS

Get into an elbow plank position. Now twist your hips to the left and then to the right. You may have the tendency to slightly raise your hips as you're twisting—avoid it!

Make sure you maintain the plank position as you're twisting your torso, and don't let either your hips go up or your body sink in.

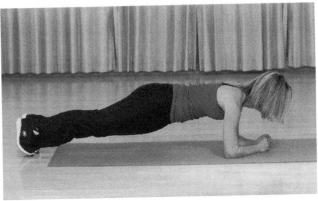

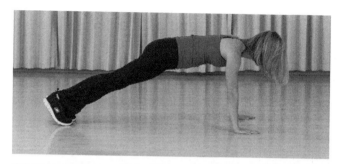

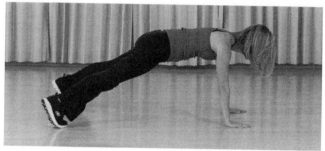

PLANK
OPEN & CLOSE

Go down into plank position. Then jump and open your legs more than hip width apart. Quickly jump again, and bring your feet together to starting position.

If jumping is hard, then just step to the sides to open your legs and then step again, one leg at a time, to bring them back together.

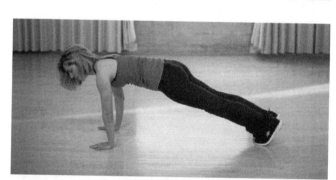

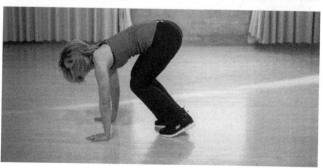

PLANK IN & OUT

Go down into plank position. With your body straight, jump forward, bringing your feet a couple of inches behind your palms. Quickly jump back to starting position and repeat.

If jumping is too hard, then just step to the front and then step to the back.

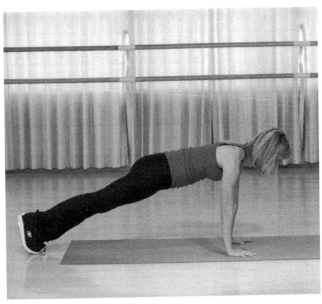

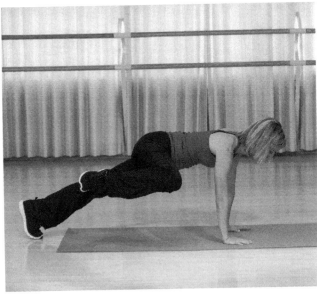

PLANK
WITH ALTERNATING
SIDE LEG

Go down into a plank position. It can either be an elbow plank or it can be a regular plank. Balancing on one leg, bend your other knee and bring your leg to the side. Then repeat for your other leg.

This is a hip-opener plank. You'll need to really work your obliques and your outer thighs in order to bring your leg to the side, high above the floor.

You may have the tendency to drop your leg down as you're bringing it to the side. Resist this urge by contracting your obliques and outer thighs. We really want those muscles to work. In FB16, we only have sixteen minutes, so for those sixteen minutes, we want to be effective and efficient. We don't want to just let time pass. We don't want to just say we worked out. Try to do your best.

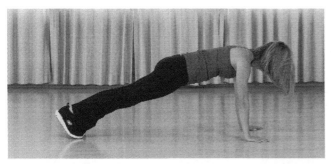

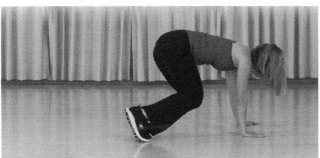

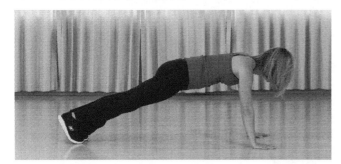

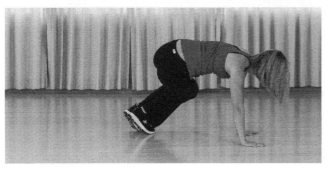

SKI ABS

Go down into plank position. Then jump and bring both feet forward and to your right. Jump again and bring your feet back to the plank position.

Then jump once more and bring your feet forward and to the left. Bring your feet back to starting position and repeat.

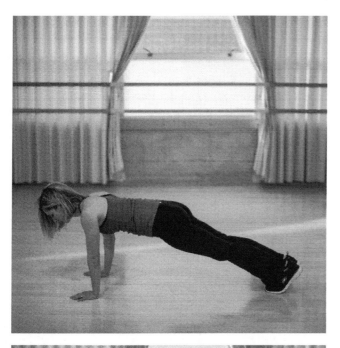

SHOULDER PLANK

Get into a plank position. Then use your shoulder blades to lift your upper body one inch. If this is hard to picture, then imagine that you're pushing against the floor, lifting your upper back up. Don't move your hips. All the motion comes from your shoulders. Then release and return to starting position.

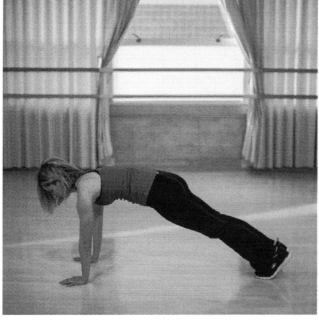

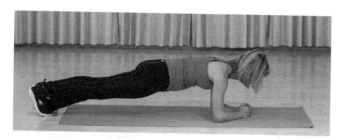

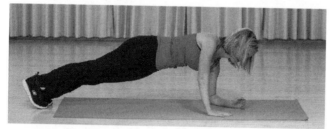

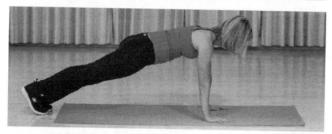

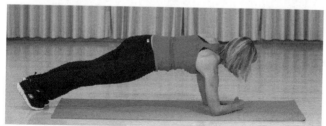

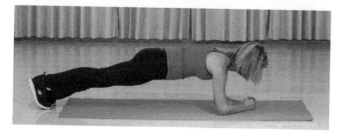

CLIMBING PLANK

In my opinion, this is the hardest variation from the plank series, but it is, oh, so worth it! Get into an elbow plank. Now straighten one arm, then the other, getting up into a regular plank position. Now climb back down to get into an elbow plank, and repeat.

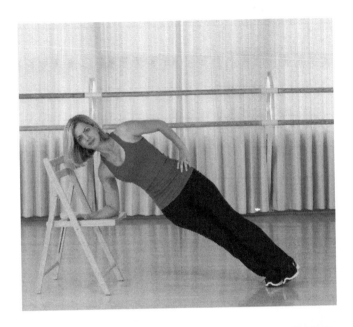

CHAIR SIDE PLANK

You'll need a chair for this one. Alternatively, you can use the arm of a sofa. Put one forearm on the chair while your body is straight in a side plank. Hold this position, and then change sides.

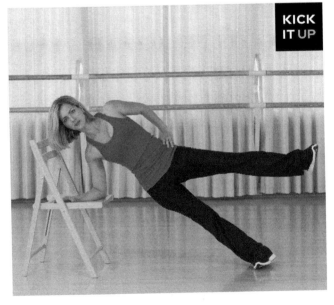

KICK IT UP

CHAIR SIDE
PLANK LIFTS

Get into a chair side plank position. Lift one leg up and then bring it back down. Then do it again for your other side.

THE C-ABS SERIES

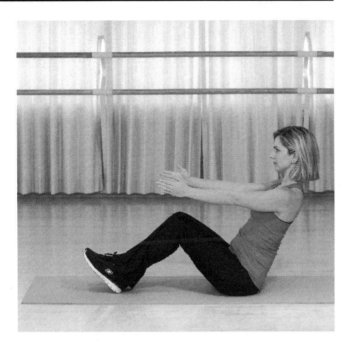

C-ABS

Sit on the mat with your knees bent and your back straight. Extend your arms to the front at shoulder level. Find your tripod of stability, which includes your two seat bones and your tailbone.

Keeping your back straight, contract your abs, and bring your torso towards the back. Feel your abs working as you go lower. The lower you go, the harder it gets.

Find the height that fits your fitness level, and start pulsing, moving your torso three inches to the front and then back.

Many people tend to arch their back while in the C position. Please avoid this tendency, or you risk injuring your lower back. Place a cushion right behind your back to get the extra support you need.

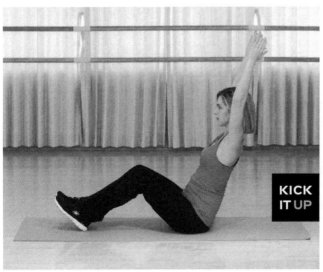

KICK IT UP

C-ABS
WITH ARMS UP

Lift your arms up, right next to your ears. Harder, huh?

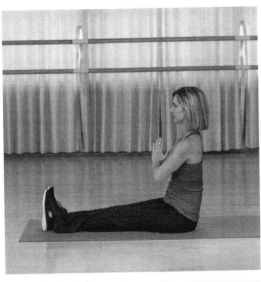

C-ABS TWISTS

Sit on the floor with your back straight and knees bent. Now straighten your knees so that your legs are completely on the floor. Keep your chest lifted and your palms together in front of your heart.

Now gradually start twisting your torso to the right and to the left while you lean back and bend your knees, getting into the classic C-abs position. Keep twisting.

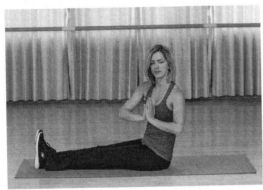

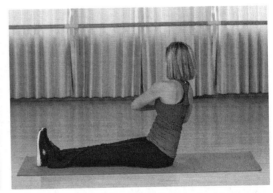

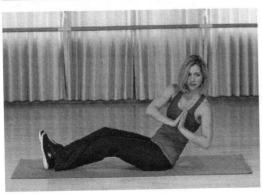

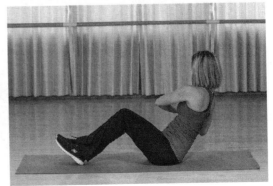

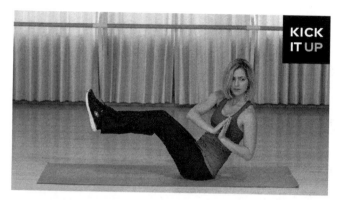

KICK IT UP

ADVANCED
C-ABS TWISTS

Lift your heels up so that your shins are parallel on the floor while you keep twisting your torso.

Want to still level it up? Straighten your legs so that your body creates a V shape. Keep twisting!

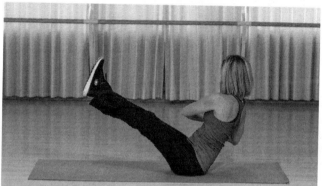

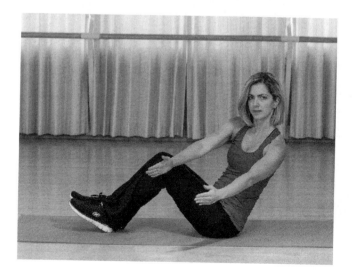

C-ABS OBLIQUE

Get into a C-abs position. Extend your arms to the front. Now twist your torso towards the right so that both your arms are on the outer side of your right leg.

Start rocking your body three inches to the back and then to the front. Feel your oblique muscles working. Once finished, repeat for the other side.

THE **FLAT BACK SERIES**

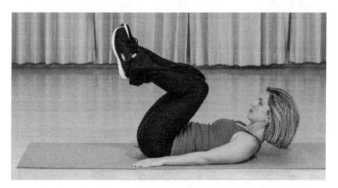

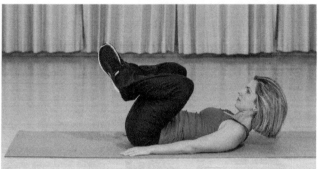

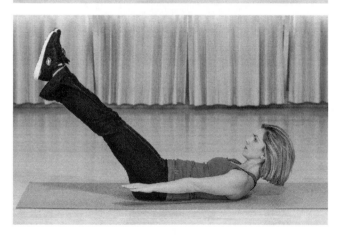

LADYBUG

Lie down on the floor with your arms next to your body. With your knees over your hips, bring your heels together with flexed feet to form a double V shape. Now raise your head and shoulder blades off the floor. Raise your arms a few inches above the floor. Keep your feet together as you straighten your legs to the front.

Now bend your knees and bring them back. Repeat. Make sure your head and arms remain lifted throughout the movement. The lower your legs when on the extended position, the harder this exercise becomes.

Make sure you keep your lower back flat on the floor as you extend your legs. Arching it ruins the form of the exercise and puts your lower back at risk. Extending your legs higher will make the exercise easier and decrease your tendency to arch your lower back.

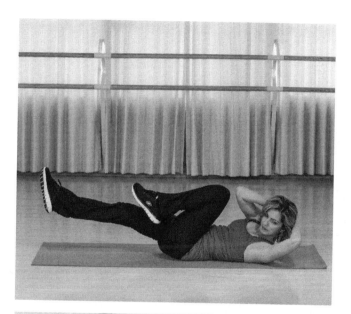

CRISS CROSS

Lie on the floor with your hands interlaced behind your head and your knees in table-top position. Extend your legs forward, and lower them down without arching your back.

Contract your abs while you lift your right shoulder off the floor and bring your left knee towards your chest. Then repeat for the other side, bringing your left elbow to almost touching your right knee.

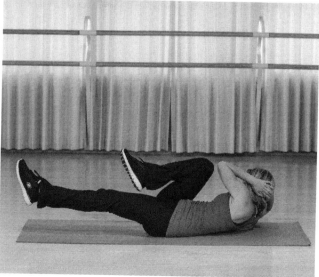

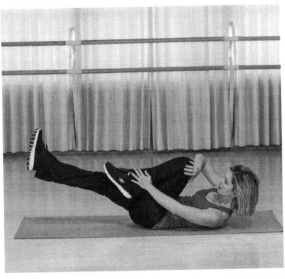

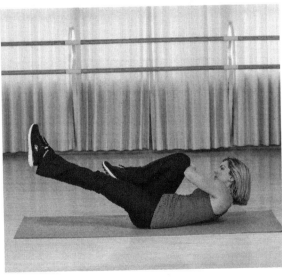

SINGLE LEG
STRETCH

Lie on the floor with your arms next to you, palms facing down. Bring your knees up on a table-top position. Now curl your head, bringing your shoulders off the mat. Draw your right knee to your chest while you extend your left leg forward.

Tap your right hand twice to the outside of the ankle of the bent leg and your left hand on the top of this knee. As you're tapping, perform two beats: bringing your shoulders and extended leg two inches higher twice. Yes, this movement requires coordination. You will be developing new motor skills.

Now switch legs, bringing your left knee to your chest and extending your right leg. Tap your left hand twice to the outside of the ankle of the bent leg and your right hand on top of this knee. Perform two beats, bringing your extended leg two inches higher, and lifting your shoulders off the floor a little more. Repeat.

This is a hard exercise to master. If you get confused, focus on one movement: start with the hand tapping, and gradually start adding the shoulder and leg movement.

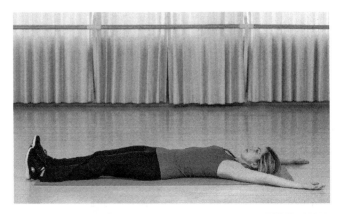

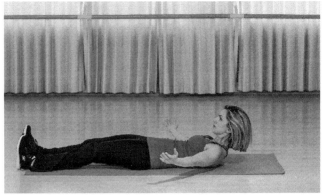

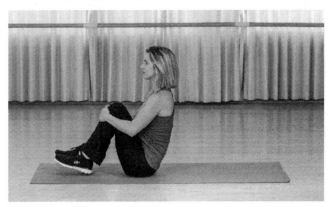

STAR ABS

An alternate name for this exercise is the star crunch. Lie down on the mat on your back with your arms open and extended above your head. Your legs are open and extended as well.

Now, with one swift motion, lift your torso up to the sitting position while you bend your knees and bring them on top of your hips. Hug your knees with your arms.

Keep your balance, and do not let your feet touch the floor. Then bring your torso and your legs back to the starting position in a controlled manner.

Pay attention to the arm movement. As you lift your torso up, your arms perform a circular movement around your body. This circular movement will engage more core muscles of your body.

THE **FOREARM SERIES**

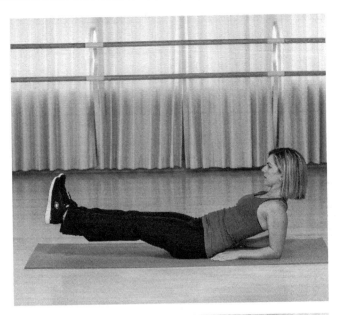

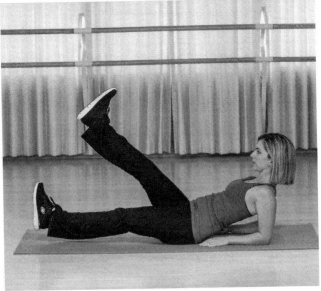

SCISSORS I

Lie on the floor with your back straight, your legs extended, and your elbows directly below your shoulders. Your palms should be flat on the floor.

  Lift both legs three inches off the floor. Push one leg higher then bring it back to the original position while you lift the other leg up. Continue alternating.

  Make sure you don't arch your lower back. If contracting your abs does not stop the arching, then lift your legs higher. The higher your legs, the easier this exercise is for your abs.

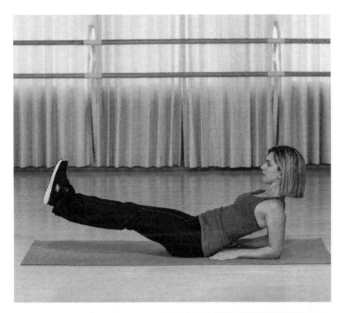

SCISSORS II

Lie on the floor with your back straight, your legs extended, and your elbows directly below your shoulders. Your palms should be flat on the floor.

Lift both legs three inches off the floor. Now open your legs without touching the floor. Then bring them back together.

Just like in Scissors I, make sure you don't arch your lower back. Also, the higher your legs, the easier this exercise is for your abs.

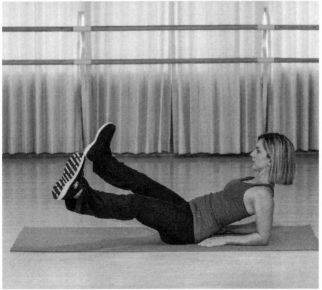

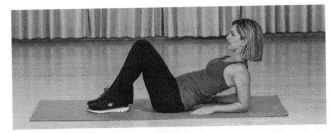

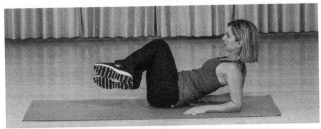

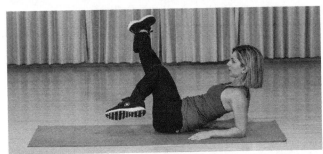

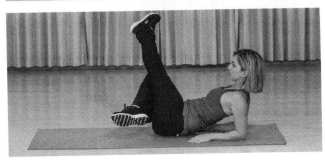

ELBOW OBLIQUE
CAN-CAN

Lie on the floor with your back straight and your elbows directly below your shoulders. Place your palms flat on the floor. Bend your knees, and bring them together on top of your hips.

Now lightly tilt your legs to the right, and then lower them to make your abs work a little more. Keeping your knees together, straighten and extend the right leg.

Now bend the right knee as you straighten your left leg. Keep alternating between legs. Contract your abs, and don't let your spine arch. Repeat for the other side.

LEGS & BUTT EXERCISES

Here are some of the best butt and legs exercises I've ever done. But doing them won't just give you lean legs and a lifted butt. You're also going to burn quite a few calories. Why? Because our legs have the biggest muscles of our bodies. The bigger the muscle, the more calories it burns. And that's why butt and leg workouts burn the most calories. Let's start melting!

THE **SQUAT AND LUNGE SERIES**

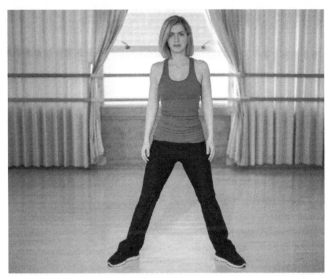

front view

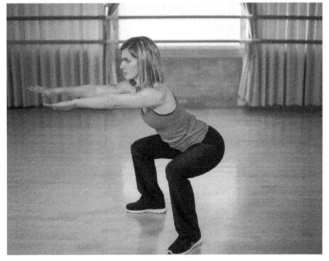

side view

SQUATS

Stand with your feet hip width apart, arms at your sides. Extend your arms at shoulder level, keep your back straight, and squat down as low as you can. Imagine you're sitting on a chair behind you.

Make sure your knees do not go in front of your toes. Push back up through your heels to starting position and repeat.

Do not over-lean or under-lean during the squat as it adds extra strain on your knee and ankle joints. Although a deep squat is considered beneficial, not everyone is capable at the beginning due to poor conditioning or due to previous injuries. So don't sweat it if you find it hard to go low. You'll get better with time.

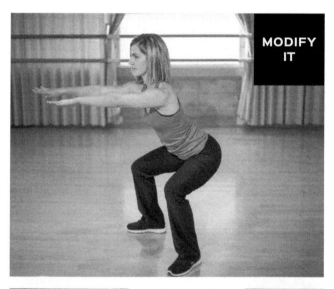

MODIFY
IT

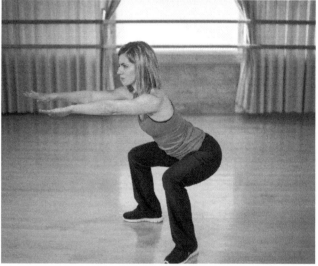

SQUAT PULSES

Bring your feet a bit more than hip width apart with your feet facing about 30 degrees out to the sides. Always maintain a straight back by pushing your chest out and by tucking your pelvis in.

Look forward, extend your arms ahead of you (to keep balance), take a deep breath, then squat down relative to your flexibility. Lower your seat down as low as you can, as if you were trying to sit on a chair behind you. Rather than coming back to the starting position right away, hold that seated squat position at the bottom as you pulse a few inches up and down for the entire exercise.

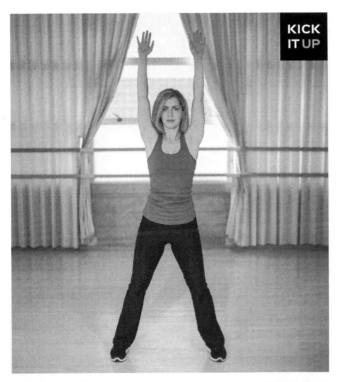

KICK
IT UP

SQUAT
TOUCH & REACH

Bring your feet a bit more than hip width apart with your feet facing about 30 degrees out to the sides. Always maintain a straight back by pushing your chest out and by tucking your pelvis in.

Look forward, extend your arms above your head, take a deep breath, then squat down. Lower your seat down as low as you can, as if you were trying to sit on a chair behind you, while at the same time lowering your hands. If you can, touch the floor with your fingertips. Come back up to starting position and repeat.

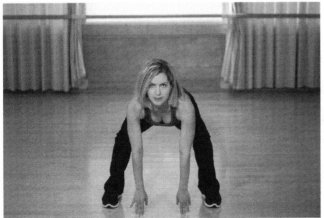

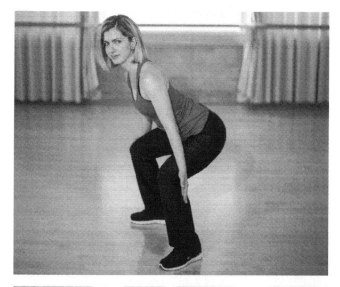

JACK SQUATS

This exercise is almost like a jumping jack, but it includes a squat. Go into a squat stance, but this time keep your legs shoulder width apart with your feet at a 45 degree angle. Instead of having your arms facing forward, they will be straddling the sides of your outer thighs with your fingers next to your knees.

Jump up with your hands straight overhead, and bring your feet together. Jump back to starting position and repeat.

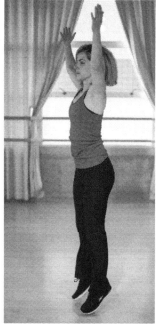
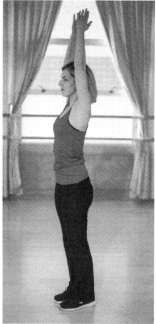

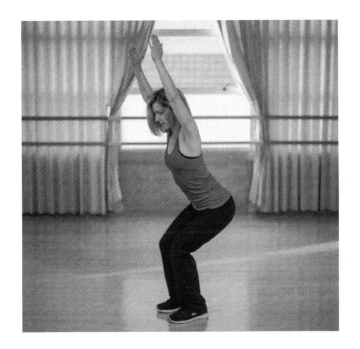

INVISIBLE CHAIR

Stand up straight with your knees and feet together. Raise your hands up in the air, push your chest out, and slowly lower your seat down, as if you're sitting on an invisible chair behind you. The lower you go, the harder this exercise becomes.

Once you reach the lowest level, hold this position. Maintain a straight back, and keep your pelvis tucked in throughout the duration of the exercise.

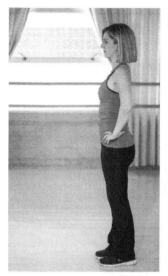
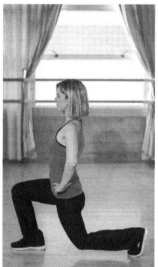
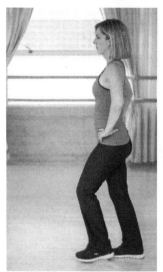
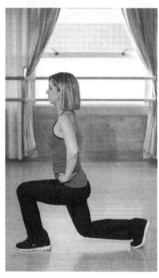

ALTERNATING
LUNGES

Stand straight with your feet together. Bringing your left heel off the floor, step forward with your right foot so that your quadriceps become parallel to the floor. Now bring yourself back to starting position with your feet together, and repeat for other leg.

As you step forward, make sure your knee does not stick out in front of your toes. The lower you bring your seat, the harder this exercise gets. It's up to you to adjust it to your fitness level.

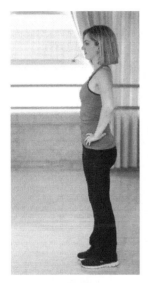
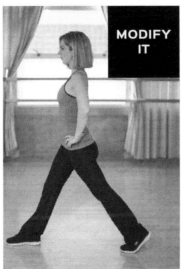

MODIFY
IT

STATIC LUNGES

Stand straight with your feet together. Step forward with your right foot so that your quadriceps become parallel to the floor.

Push yourself back up, creating a triangle shape with your legs, and then bend your knees again to repeat the lunge.

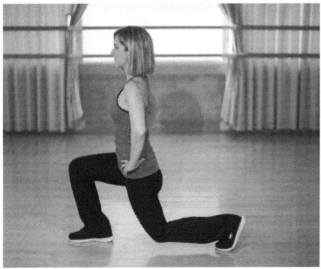

THE **FLOOR SERIES**

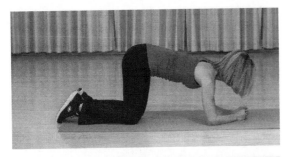

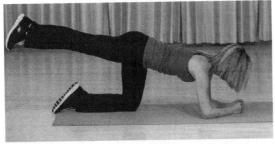

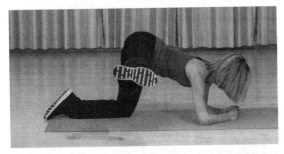

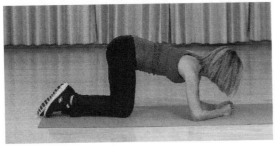

GLOBE GLUTES

Get on the floor with your knees below your hips and your elbows below your shoulders. Now extend one leg to the back. Then contract your glutes to bring it up to hip level and use your core muscles to rotate this leg to the side.

Open your hips as much as possible, and don't let your leg drop. Then bend your knee and bring your leg back to starting position. Repeat for the other leg.

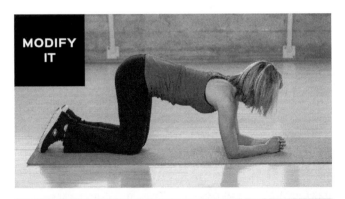

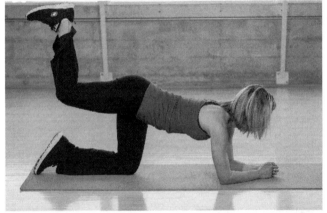

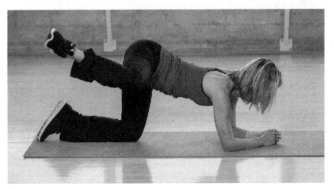

HALF
GLOBE GLUTES

Get on the floor with your knees below your hips and your elbows below your shoulders. Keep your back straight, making sure you're not arching your back.

Now with your foot flexed, lift one knee up at hip level. Now rotate to the side, opening your hips as much as possible and holding that leg up. Bring it back to starting position and repeat for the other leg. By rotating your leg, you're working all the tiny muscles in your butt, giving your behind the nice, lifted shape you want it to have.

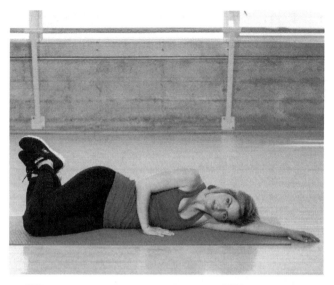

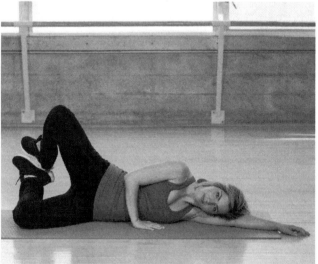

CLAMS

This is a perfect exercise for your hips with a high preventative value against the hip-related perils of old age.

Lie on your side, resting your head on your hand. Place your upper hand in front of your belly for support. Bring your feet and knees together, keeping your legs bent.

Now lift your feet off the floor. Slowly raise your top knee then bring it back down and repeat until the time is up. Repeat for your other side.

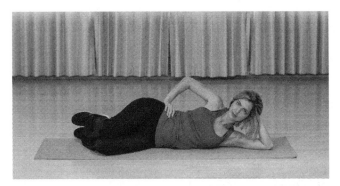

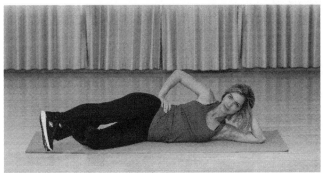

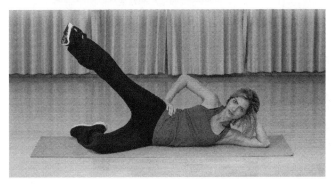

DIAGONAL
LEG LIFTS

Lie on your side, resting your head on your hand, with your feet and knees together. Place your upper hand in front of your belly for balance. Keep your lower leg slightly bent while you straighten your upper leg and slightly lift it off the floor.

Now bring your leg to a 30 degree angle. Rotate it so that your toes point to the floor. Lift your leg up, and then bring it down without touching the floor. Repeat until the time is up, and then repeat for other side.

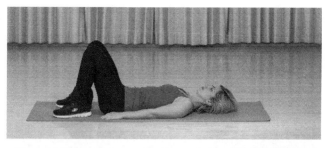

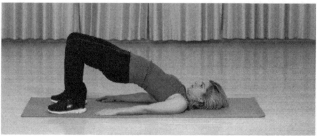

SHOULDER BRIDGE

Lie on your back with your knees bent and feet hip width apart. Your arms should be right next to your body.

Contract your abs and glutes as you push your bottom straight up, creating a diagonal line with your body, then return to starting position.

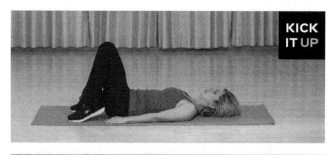

KICK
IT UP

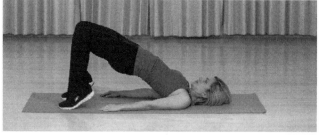

SHOULDER BRIDGE
ON TOES

Lay supine to the floor. Place your arms flat next to you on the floor. Now lift your heels up, until you are on your toes.

Lift your seat off the floor. Return to starting position and repeat.

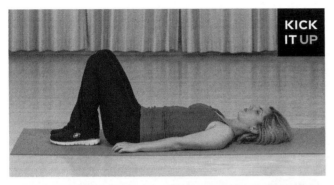

KICK
IT UP

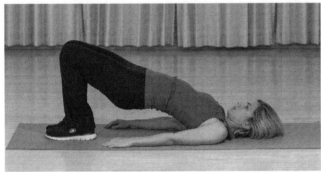

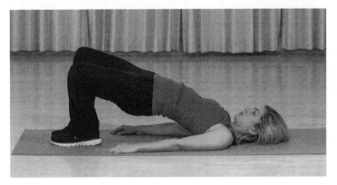

SHOULDER BRIDGE
OPEN–CLOSE

Lie on your back with your knees bent and your feet next to each other. Your arms should be right next to your body. You can be on your toes, or you can put your feet flat on the mat.

Lift your seat up, keeping your knees and feet together. Now open your knees, creating a diamond shape, and then bring them back together. Repeat.

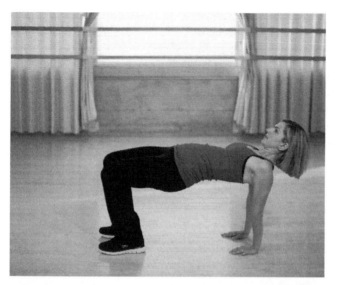

TABLE KICKS

Imagine yourself becoming a human table: With your back facing the floor, knees bent at 90 degrees and arms with flat hands left straight under your shoulders.

Keep your torso linear by lifting your hips up till straight. As fast as possible, extend your leg and then bring it back down while you extend the other.

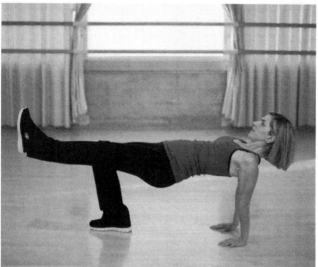

THE **CHAIR-ASSISTED EXERCISES**

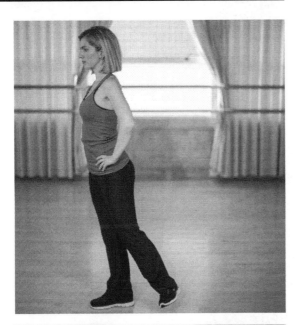

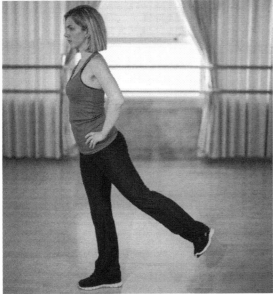

FIGURE SKATER

With your feet together, move your leg to the back. Rotate it so that your toes point to a 30 degree angle. Keep the supporting leg locked in place.

Now push your other leg three inches above the floor and bring it back down without touching the floor.

Do not lean overly forward, and do not turn your hips to the side; instead, keep them square. Once finished, repeat for your other leg.

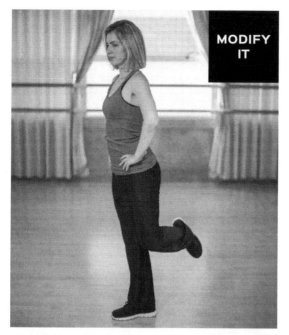

MODIFY IT

HALF
FIGURE SKATER

Stand with both feet together. Now turn one foot on the diagonal, bend that knee 45 degrees, and lift it up as high as you can.

Now push your leg three inches higher. Rather than coming back to the starting position right away, hold your leg up as you pulse a few inches up and down for the entire exercise. Repeat for your other leg.

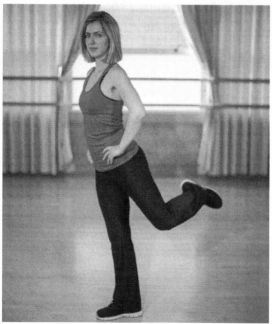

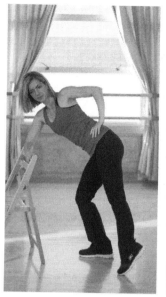
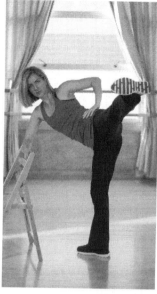

CHAIR SIDE LIFTS

This is a great love-handle killer—you know, that jiggly stuff on the sides of your body that you could do without?

Use the back of a chair or sofa for support. You can also use a table or any surface that is at least waist high.

With your back straight, rest your elbow on the chair and lift one leg to the side, keeping it straight. Now touch the floor with your toes, and then lift back up. Repeat.

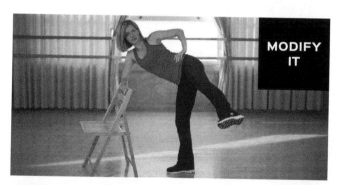

MODIFY IT

CHAIR SIDE PULSES

Instead of doing the whole movement with your leg and touching the floor, bring your leg three inches down. Then lift back up and repeat.

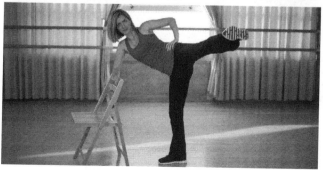

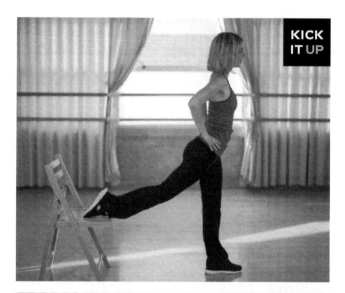

KICK IT UP

CHAIR LUNGES

Definitely one of the hardest lunges you can do. As the name suggests, you'll need a chair for this one. Step away from the chair. Now lift one leg up, and put one foot on top of it. Do not let your hips turn, and instead keep them square.

Now bend your other leg to go down into a lunge. Then push yourself back to starting position and repeat until the time is up. Repeat for the other leg.

If you find that your knee goes in front of your toes as you go down, then adjust your position by stepping farther away from the chair and repeat till you can do the lunge properly. If you find it hard to balance, then hold on to a piece of furniture or a wall.

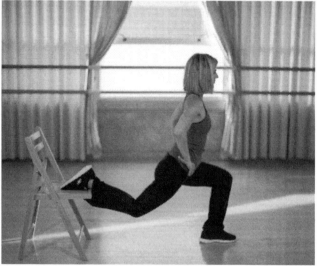

THE JUMPS

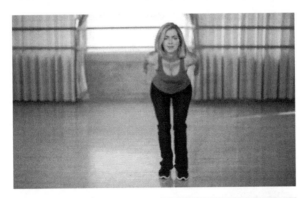

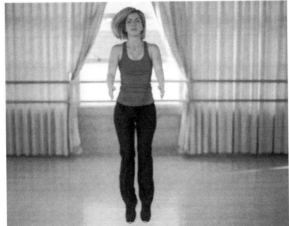

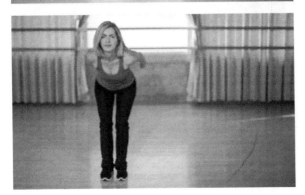

SKI JUMPS

Bring your feet together, and slightly bend your knees as if you're skier. Lean forward and move your arms to the back.
 Now jump to the side while straightening your body and bringing your arms to the front. Land softly, bringing your arms to the back, and jump back to starting position.

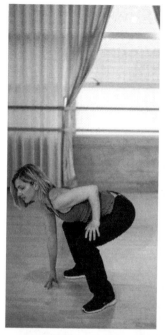
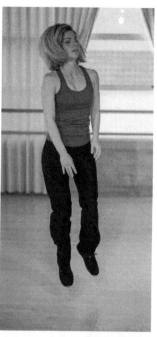
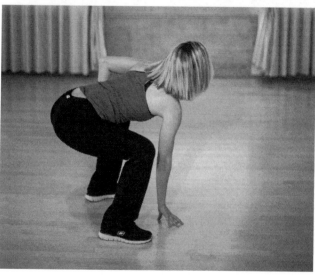

SNOWBOARDER'S JUMPS

This is one of the harder squat variations. You may also hear it called "Snowboarder's Squats." With your feet more than hip width apart, squat down, resting one hand on your leg and touching the floor with the other hand. Now jump 180 degrees and land (softly) squatted down, touching the floor with the same arm.

Again, if touching the floor is hard, then don't push yourself to squat low. Also, make sure you land softly. In Greece, we say, "Do not land like a bag of potatoes." Exactly. Do not land on the ground making a huge sound and risking knee injuries. Control the movement, and land on the ground softly, as if you were a cat.

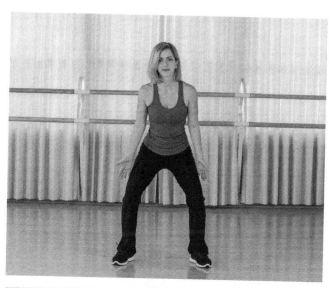

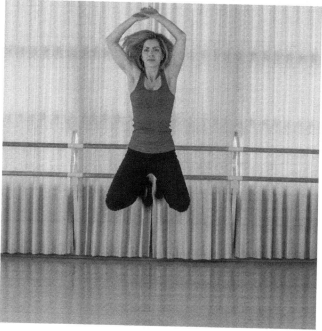

DIAMOND JUMPS

This is an amazing fat-burning exercise that will both strengthen your muscles and get your heart rate up. You might also hear it called "Diamond Squats."

Start with your feet more than hip width apart. Now squat down with your arms slightly bent and your hands just above your knees. Jump up while you bring your feet together and while you raise your arms high above your head, bringing your palms together.

Land softly in a squat position with your hands right above your knees and repeat.

If jumping is hard, then perform an easier squat variation like the "Squat Touch & Reach".

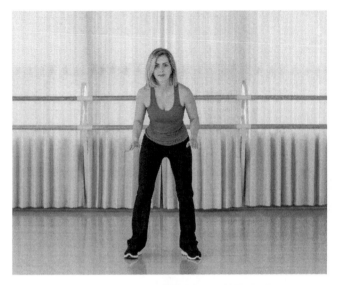

POWER JUMPS

If you're looking to sculpt your legs—and fast—then look no further. Power jumps (else known as "Power Squats") will do it for you.

Get into a squat position with your feet shoulder width apart and your elbows bent with your forearms parallel to the floor. Now jump high above the ground, bringing your knees up to hip level. While in the air, clap your hands on your knees. Land softly and repeat.

If jumping is difficult, then perform an easier squat variation like the squat pulses.

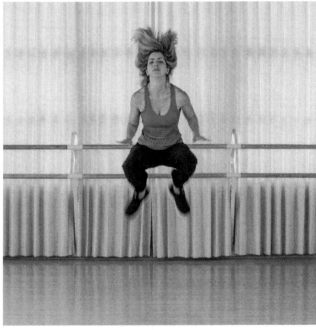

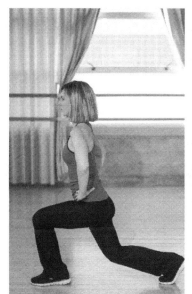 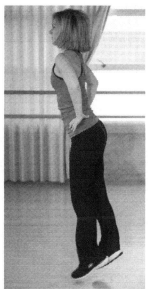 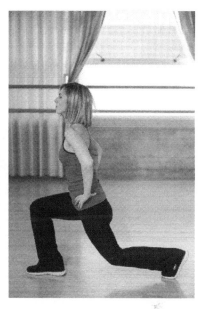

JUMPING LUNGES

Your heart rate will really go up with this one. Get into a lunge position with both knees bent. Keep your back straight.
 Now jump up while you alternate legs mid-air. Land softly and repeat.

UPPER BODY
EXERCISES

Now, if you are a guy and you're reading this, then I'm sure you get why working your arms, back, shoulders, and chest is important. But if you are a woman, I know we women tend to sometimes neglect the upper part of our bodies in favor of "juicier" parts. So let me explain to you why exactly upper body should not be neglected.

First of all, you will have better-looking arms. Your arms and shoulders are going to look better or your shoulders will look better when you wear a strapless shirt. Second, strong upper body will also have a "functional" difference in your life. Say you need to get a baby into a car seat; you'll be using your upper body muscles to make this out-and-into-the-car movement happen. It's not uncommon for new moms to get lower back injuries from this movement. With a strong upper body, you'll be protecting yourself from such problems.

Finally, a strong upper body will improve your posture, effectively reducing your risk for lower back pain. But better posture is not just about avoiding pain; it's also about better looks. I've already discussed how I always find it strange that people may whine about those extra five pounds when they could easily look like they're five pounds thinner by walking with a straighter posture!

Now here's what you will need to do the exercises in this section. I suggest you use two sets of weights, a lighter and a heavier one. I use the lighter one for shoulder-work and the heavier one for everything else. Take note of what the number on your dumbbells is. If the number is too low, then this workout might actually feel quite easy. So if these exercises feel easy, then you know you need to increase the number on your weights.

Now, if you have no weights available, then be creative. You can, for example, use two bottles of water—just keep them full. I want the bottles to be full because if you're lifting, say, a half-empty bottle, then the water will be moving around as you're lifting the bottle, altering the exercise. Go for a full bottle instead, and make sure the lid is securely shut. You don't want water spilled all over!

If you don't have bottles, then you could grab a book. Alternatively, you could use a backpack filled with as many books as you can lift. Now enough with the instructions. It's time to get into action!

THE **PUSH-UPS**

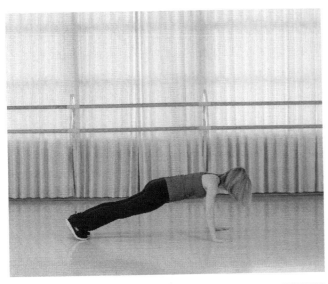

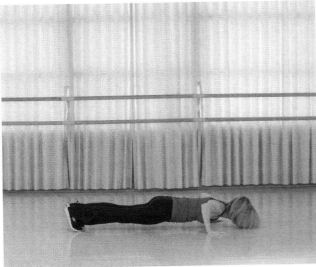

CLASSIC PUSH-UP

Get into a plank position with your palms underneath your shoulders and your feet together.

Now bend your elbows and lower your body until your chin or torso is almost touching the floor. Push yourself up to starting position and repeat.

Make sure that you're neither sticking your butt out nor letting your hips sag down. This is not proper push-up form. Also, take care that your body remains in a perfectly straight plank position both when you're going down and when you're pushing yourself up.

Finally, pay attention. Are you lowering your body as close to the floor as possible? Or, are you only pretending you're doing push-ups? Don't take C for effort, give it your all!

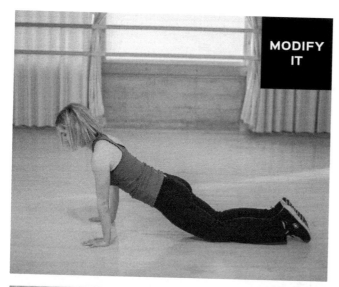

MODIFY IT

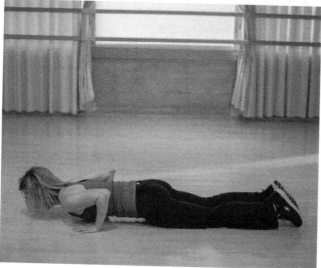

HALF PUSH-UP

If you're not ready for the full push-up yet, then no worries. The half push-up comes to the rescue.

Just like in the regular push-up, get into a plank position with your palms beneath your shoulders. Now touch your knees on the floor.

Lower your body down until your torso or chin almost touches the floor. Then push your body back up and repeat.

Here's a hint that can slightly change how this exercise feels. The closer your upper arms are to your body, the harder push-ups become and the more you work your triceps, the muscles at the back of your upper arms.

If, instead, your arms are open, with your palms not beneath your shoulders but in parallel to them, your chest muscles get worked more and the exercise feels easier. Choose the arm position that fits your needs the best.

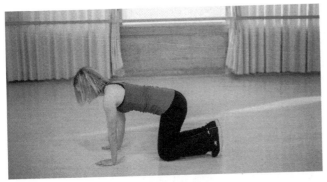

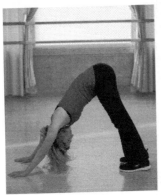

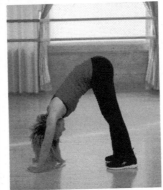

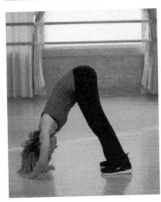

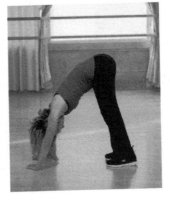

V PUSH-UP

Get on the floor in a table position with your palms underneath your shoulders and your knees below your hips. Your back should be straight and your pelvis tucked in.

Now straighten your legs, creating a reverse V shape with your body. Walk your feet one or two steps towards your palms, and turn your palms a little so that they face each other. Bend your elbows, effectively lowering your body, and then push yourself back up to return to starting position.

If you don't yet have the flexibility to straighten your legs, then no worries. As long as you keep your back straight, it's okay if your legs are slightly bent instead of perfectly straight. Flexibility will come with time and practice.

THE **SHOULDER & BACK EXERCISES**

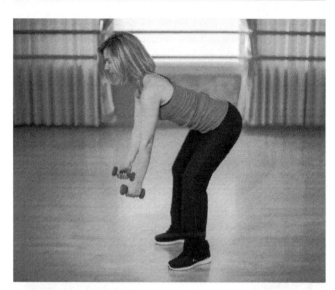

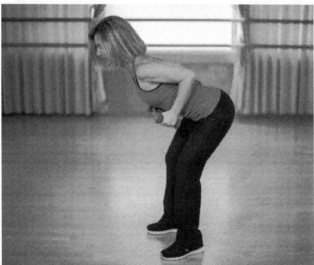

ROWS

Get your heavier sets of weights. It's time to build a long, lean back, stand taller, and have a better posture.

With your feet hip width apart, keep your back straight as you bend forward to a 45-degree angle. With your palms facing in, let your arms hang down, but don't let your shoulders hang. Instead, keep your shoulders back and in place, and only let your arms follow the pull of gravity.

Now contract your back muscles and lift both weights up, bringing your upper arms in line with your torso. Keep your elbows as close to your body as you can. Then, in a slow controlled motion, extend your arms again and repeat.

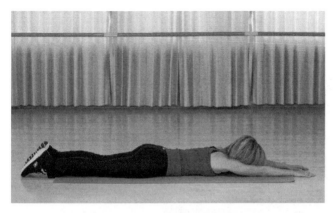

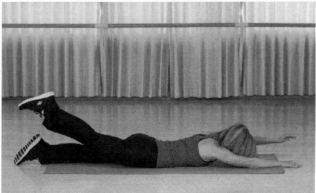

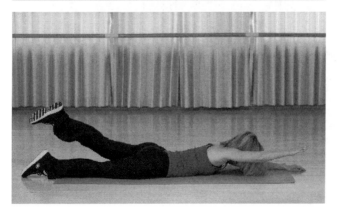

SUPERMAN

Lie belly down on your mat with your forehead slightly above the floor. Your arms and legs are extended.

Now raise one arm along with the opposite leg, then bring them back down while you lift your opposite arm and leg.

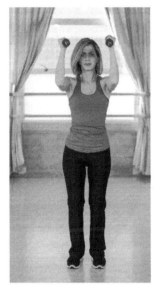 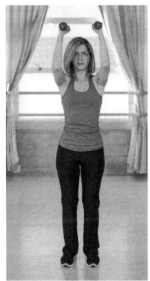

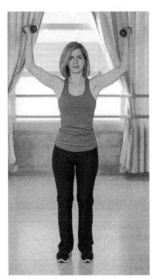

SHOULDER PULSES

Grab your lighter sets of weights, and stand with your feet hip width apart, keeping your back straight. Bend your knees just a little.

With your palms facing each other, bend your arms to a 90-degree angle and raise your elbows slightly below shoulder level. Now begin lifting the weights in small upward pulses.

Make sure you keep your shoulders down all throughout this exercise.

WIDER
SHOULDER PULSES

This is the exact same exercise as the regular shoulder pulses but with a back fat burning twist. The main difference is the position of your elbows.

Both hands are turned towards your body. Both elbows are bent in a 90-degree angle, but instead of having your elbows right in front of your shoulders, your elbows are opened more than shoulder-level width apart. In this position, perform small upward pulses.

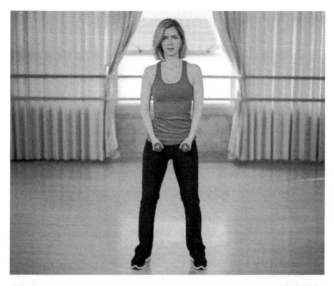

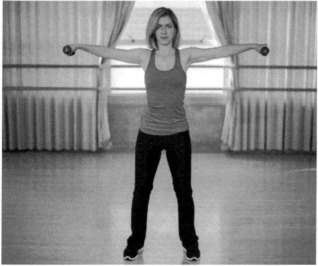

SHOULDER
LATERAL LIFTS

Beautiful, sculpted shoulders—that's exactly what you'll get with this exercise.

Get your lighter set of weights. With your legs hip width apart and knees slightly bent, keep your back straight and your pelvis tucked in. Turn the dumbbells so that the palms are facing each other, and slightly bend your elbows.

Now lift your arms laterally, bringing them up in line with your shoulders. Then lower them down to starting position.

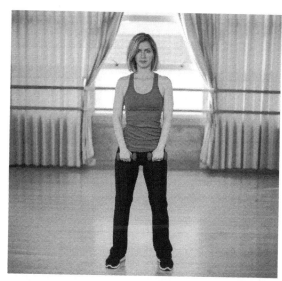

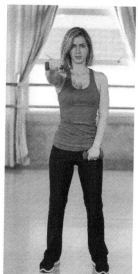

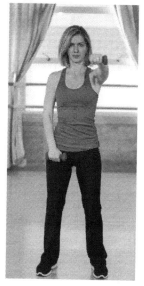

SHOULDER
FRONT LIFTS

Start by standing with your feet shoulder width apart and the torso in an upright position with a dumbbell in each hand. Turn the dumbbells so that the palms are facing your thighs and your elbows are slightly bent.

Keeping your arm just slightly bent, raise your right arm in front of you until the dumbbell is directly in front of your shoulder. Then lower this arm down as you bring the other arm up.

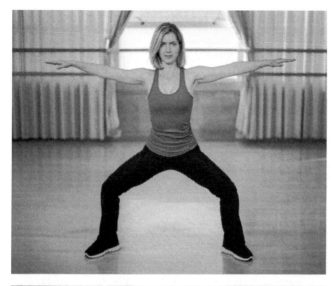

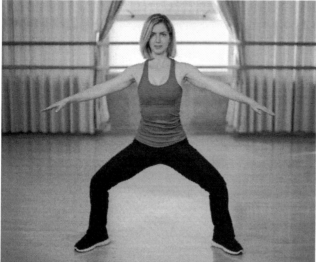

ARM WINGS

Time to spread your wings! With your legs more than hip width apart and your back straight, lower your seat down and get into a squat position. Now straighten your arms and raise them up laterally on shoulder level.

Keeping your body in a squat position, push your arms up and then back down, performing small upward pulses. Imagine your arms are your wings and you're learning to fly. Keep pulsing with your arms until time is up.

THE **ARM EXERCISES**

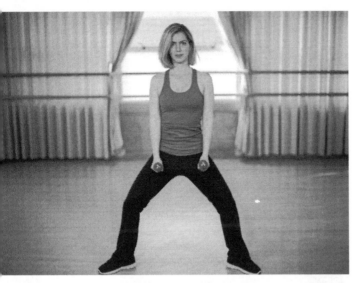

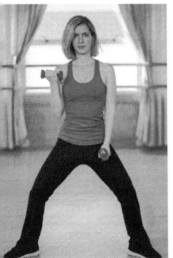
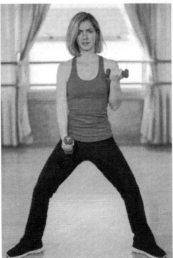

BICEP CURLS
ON HALF SQUAT

Now let's pump up those guns! Get your heavier sets of weights.

Stand straight with your feet more than hip width apart and knees bent in a squat position. Your arms should be right next to your body with your palms facing in.

Keep your upper arms glued to your body as you bring one forearm up next to your shoulder and as you rotate your forearm so that your palm faces your shoulder. Then bring this forearm down to starting position as you bring the other forearm up.

Keep your pelvis tucked in at all times, and never let your shoulders hang. Instead, keep your posture long and straight.

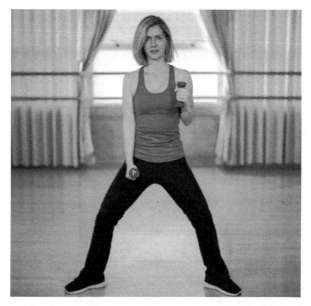

HAMMERS
ON HALF SQUAT

Another gun-enhancing exercise! This is just like Bicep Curls, but it works your muscles from a different angle.

Instead of curling your forearm as you bring it up, you lift your forearm up exactly as it is. Your palms keep facing in at all times.

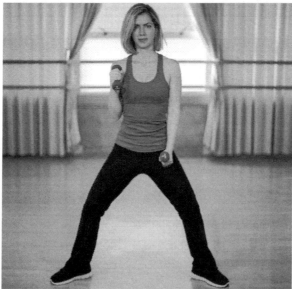

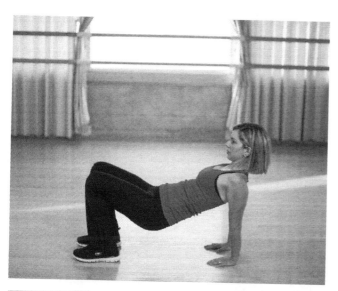

TRICEP DIPS

Sit on the floor with your knees bent, your feet flat on the floor, and your arms a few inches behind you, palms on the floor pointing forward.

Now contract your triceps, the muscles at the back of your arms, to extend your arms and push your hips above the floor. Then bend your elbows without touching the floor with your seat. Repeat bending and straightening your elbows to develop the leanest arms you can imagine.

Keep your shoulders back and your chest lifted at all times.

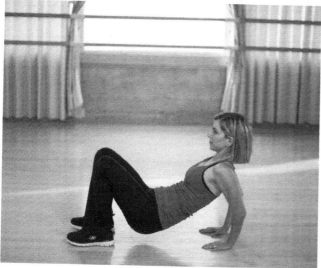

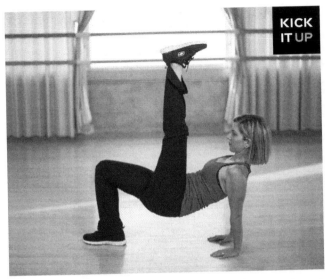

KICK IT UP

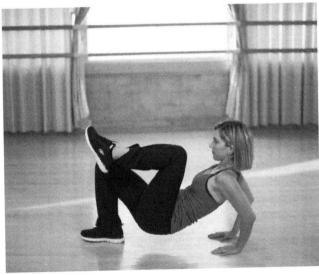

TRICEP CAN-CAN

Now let's take it one level up. With this exercise, we'll give your triceps a harder time, plus your abdominals will start working too.

Get into a tricep dips position with your palms a few inches behind you, knees bent, feet flat on the floor, and palms pointing forward. Now lift one leg straight up in the air.

As you bend your elbows to perform a dip, you also bend your knee, bringing your foot in line with your knee. Now straighten your arms to return to starting position while simultaneously extending your leg. Repeat until time is up, and then repeat for other leg.

This exercise needs a little practice to master coordinating your arms and leg, but the result is totally worth it!

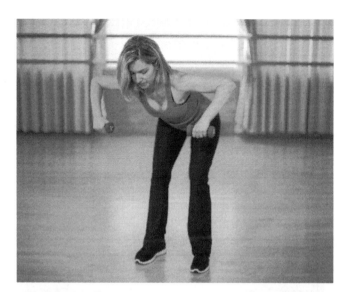

SCARECROWS

With your feet hip width apart, keep your back straight as you bend forward to a 45-degree angle.

Bend your elbows, and bring them in line with your shoulders. Your palms should be facing behind you.

Now extend your arms, pushing the weights up. Then bend your elbows back to a 90-degree angle and repeat.

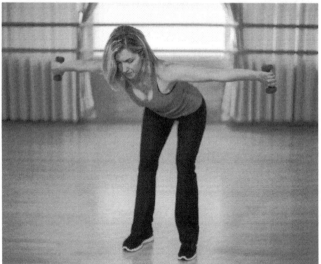

BALANCE EXERCISES

Balance exercises don't just work the body; they also work the mind. Balancing takes time, it takes commitment, and most importantly, it takes focus. You'll find it easier to keep your balance while exercising if you look at a specific spot ahead of you the whole time and avoid taking your gaze away from it. If you find yourself struggling with balance, it's okay. I'm also not perfect at it, and that's all right. The goal is progress, not perfection. Your goal is to practice a little more with every workout. It's only a matter of time—exercises that were once impossible to do without the (balancing) help of a chair or a wall will become a piece of cake. Let's get started!

$\rightarrow$

THE **LOWER BODY EXERCISES**

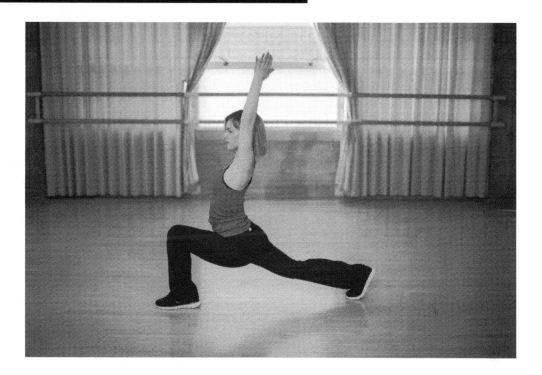

HIGH LUNGE POSE

Stand straight with your feet together. Now take a big step to the front. Both of your feet should point straight ahead.
  While keeping your back leg straight, bend your front knee to go down into a deep lunge.

Then straighten your arms, interlace your fingers, and bring your arms up next to your ears.
  Hold this position. Keep your chest lifted and make sure your hips are square at all times.

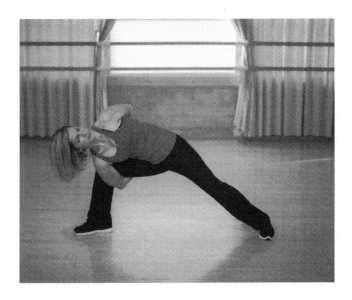

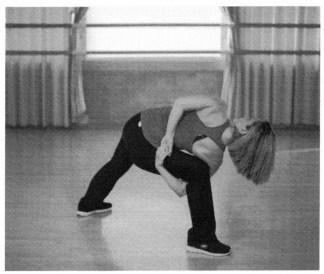

SIDE ANGLE POSE

Stand straight with your feet together. With your right leg, take a big step to the front. Rotate your back foot so that it points to a 30- or 45-degree angle. Bend your front knee to go into a deep lunge.

Now lower your torso so that it's in line with your front leg. Twist your torso, and look up as you place your right arm underneath your right leg and bring your left leg behind your back. Try to bind your hands together or catch your left wrist with your right hand. Hold this pose.

This pose needs a bit of practice to master and get the arm movement, but again, it's worth it. You're going to feel muscles you didn't even know you had!

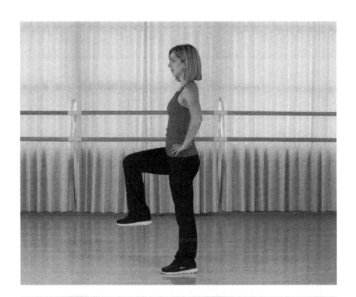

BALANCE WARRIOR

Stand straight on one leg while you lift the other knee in line with your hips. Place your palms on your waist. Find your balance.

In a controlled movement, lean your torso forward to a 90-degree angle while you bring your bent leg to the back and straighten it. Once you're ready, return to starting position, and repeat until the time is up. Then repeat for the other leg.

This exercise will be easier if instead of trying to do the whole 90-degree movement, you lean to a smaller 45-degree angle. Master the 45-degree angle first, and then getting to 90 degrees will be much easier.

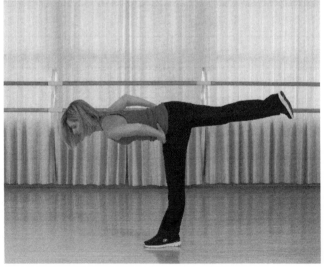

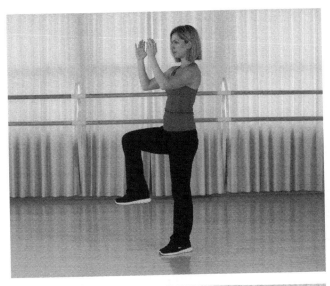

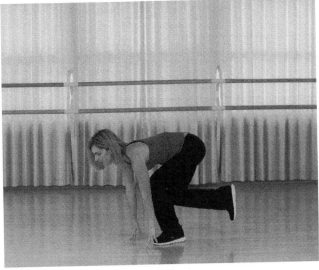

SPRINTER'S SQUAT

Stand straight, and lift your right knee in line with your hips. Find your balance. Bring your hands up as if you were a boxer.

Now bend your left knee until your thigh is parallel to the floor, and touch your left foot with your hands. Do not put your right foot on the floor to help with balance; instead, use your muscles. Go back to starting position, and repeat until time is up. Then change legs.

If actually touching the floor is hard, then don't go that low. Instead, go as low as you can. As you get stronger, you'll be able to bend your knee more and ultimately touch the floor with your hands. Don't try to force yourself to touch the floor if you are not yet ready to do it.

Finally, as with all squats, make sure your knee does not go in front of your toes.

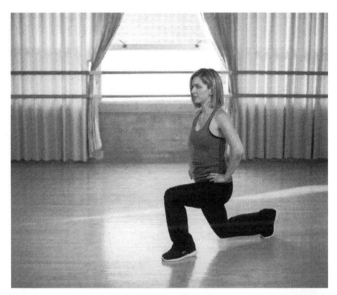

REVERSE LUNGE
AND KICK

Stand straight with your feet together. With your right leg, step back into a lunge.

Then press on the floor with your left foot as you bring your body back to starting position. Instead of touching the floor with your right foot, lift your right knee up in line with your hips.

If you can, straighten your right leg into a big kick. Then get back into the reverse lunge position and repeat. Once finished, repeat for the other side.

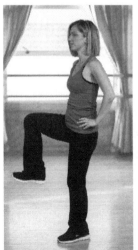

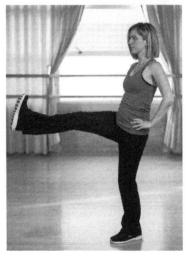

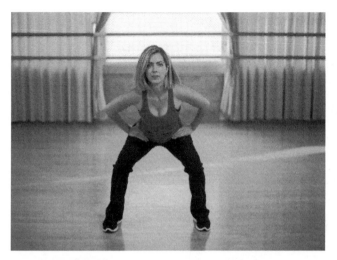

SQUAT AND BACK
LEG STRAIGHT

Stand straight with your legs more than hip width apart. Squat down. Then balance your weight on one leg as you bring the other foot right next to your balancing foot, slightly touching the floor.

Now straighten this leg as you push it back. Make sure you keep your hips square as you push your leg back.

Now bring your back leg to the front, again slightly touching the floor, and then open it to the side as you get back into the starting squatting position. Repeat the movement until time is up, and then repeat for the other leg.

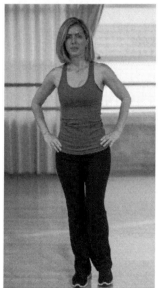

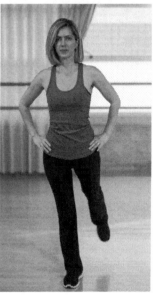

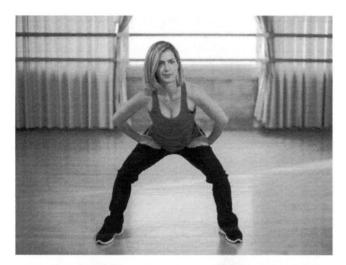

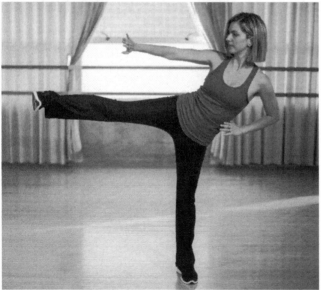

SQUAT AND SIDE
LEG STRAIGHT

This is the kick-butt magician exercise. Imagine you're a magician throwing a fireball to the enemy while kicking them in the belly. Wow, you're cool!

Here's how to make it happen. Stand straight with your legs more than hip width apart. Squat down, then balance your weight on one leg, keeping it slightly bent, while you straighten one arm in line with your shoulders for balance.

As you balance on one leg, quickly straighten your other leg and bring it up to the side in line with your hips (or higher if you want to kick the enemy in the face rather than the belly). Repeat until time is up, and then repeat for the other leg.

THE ABS EXERCISES

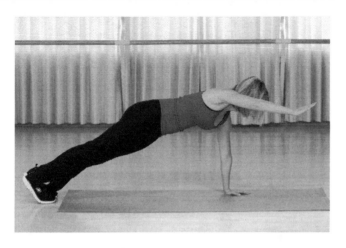

PLANK
WITH ARM UP

Get down to a classic elbow or plank position. Slowly lift one arm up. Hold this position then repeat for the other arm.

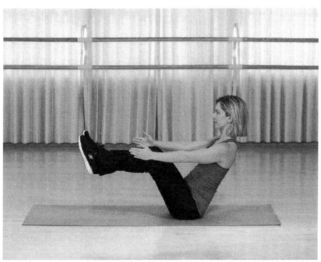

C-ABS BALANCE

Lift your feet up so that your shins are parallel to the floor. Find your balance and hold this position.

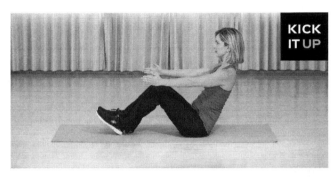

KICK
IT UP

C-ABS WITH

STRAIGHT LEGS

This is a harder C-abs variation. Get into a C-abs position, and lift your feet up so that your shins are parallel to the floor.

Now straighten your legs up so that your body creates a V shape. Hold this position.

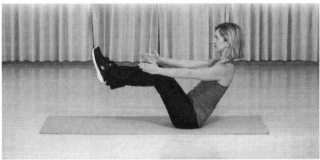

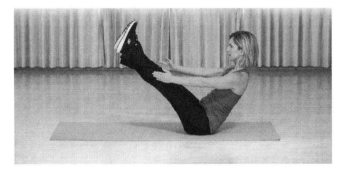

QUEEN BURPEES

Yes, I have a separate section for burpees. Why? Because burpees are such an effective exercise, you could actually do a whole 16-minute workout with just burpees. They are the ultimate total-body exercise. They work each and every muscle of your body, all while getting your heart rate up. That's why I call them the queen of exercises. Enjoy!

THE **EXERCISES**

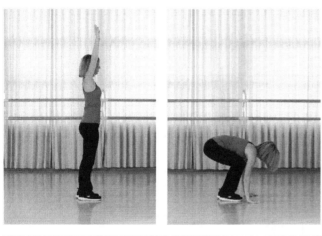

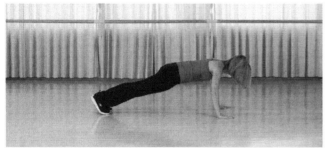

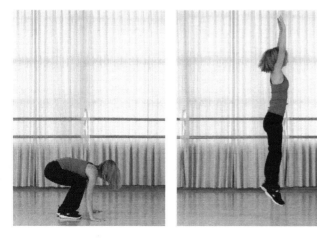

JUMPING BURPEES

Start in a standing position with your back straight and your arms straight up in the air.

Squat down, touching the floor with your hands. Put your weight on your hands as you jump back into a regular plank.

As you go into the plank, do not let your hips sag down or be raised up. Now jump forward, bringing your feet just before your palms, and then jump up as high as you can, extending your arms up in the air.

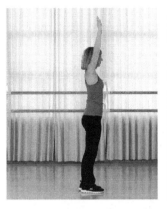

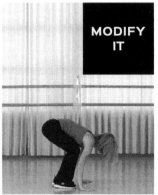

MODIFY IT

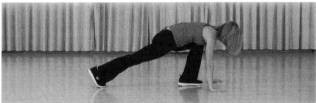

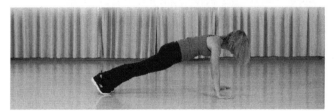

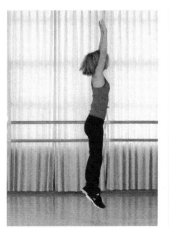

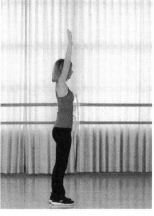

SOLDIER PLANK

Many people find it difficult to jump to the back. If this is you, then opt for the soldier plank instead of the jumping burpees.

Start in a standing position with your back straight and your arms straight up in the air. Now squat down, touching the floor with your hands.

Put your weight on your hands as you step back one leg at a time into a regular plank. Then step forward, bringing both feet behind your palms, and jump up. Land softly and repeat.

The secret of this exercise is to develop speed, and step both back and forward fast—just like an agile soldier would.

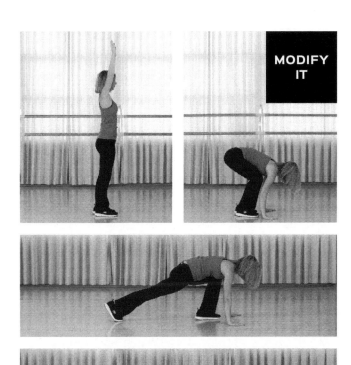

MODIFY IT

MODIFIED BURPEES

Guess what? If you don't want to do any jumps, then you can completely modify burpees to make it happen.

Start in a standing position with your back straight and your arms straight up in the air. Now squat down, touching the floor with your hands.

Put your weight on your hands as you step back one leg at a time into a regular plank. Then step forward, bringing both feet behind your palms, and stand up, with your arms straight up in the air.

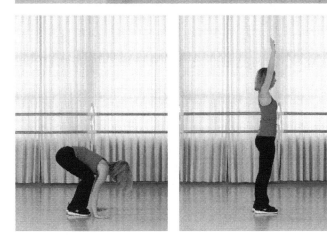

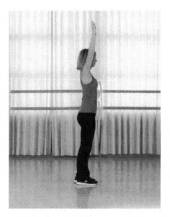
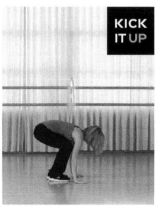

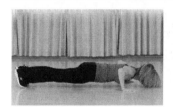
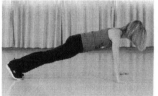

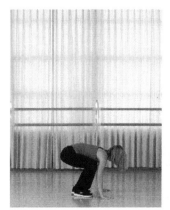
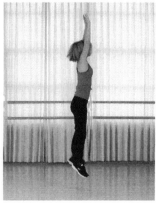

FULL JUMPING BURPEES

Now that's a burpee with a push-up. Start in a standing position with your back straight and your arms straight up in the air. Now squat down, touching the floor with your hands.

Put your weight on your hands as you jump back into a regular plank. Perform a push-up.

Jump forward, bringing your feet just before your palms, and then jump up high in the air with your arms extended above your head. Land softly and repeat.

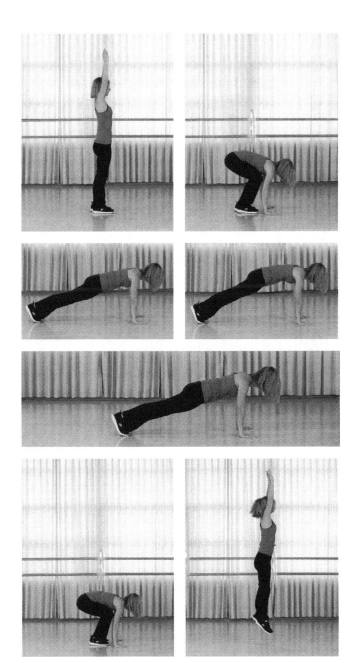

SHOULDER BURPEES

Start off in a standing position with your arms extended above your head. Jump back into the plank. Then use your shoulder blades to lift your upper body up one inch.

If this is hard to picture, then imagine that you're pushing against the floor, lifting your upper back up. Don't move your hips. All the motion comes from your shoulders. Then release and return to the plank position.

Jump forward and finish by either jumping up, or if you want to have it easier, standing back up, with your arms straight up in the air.

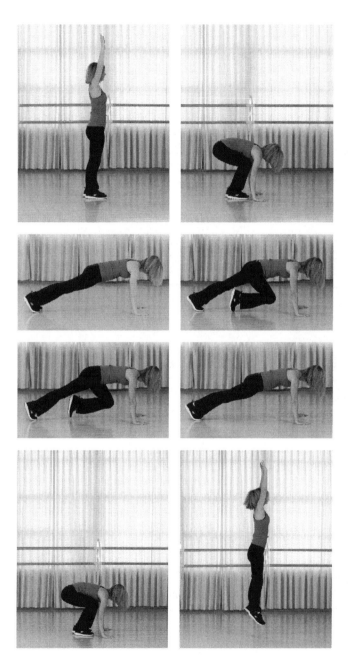

BURPEES WITH
MOUNTAIN CLIMBERS

In the "full" variation we added a push-up. In this one, we'll be adding mountain climbers right after you get into a plank.

Start off with a standing position with your arms extended above your head. Jump back into the plank. Then perform two mountain climbers by bringing each knee to your chest twice.

Then jump forward and finish by either jumping up, or if you want to make it easier, standing back up.

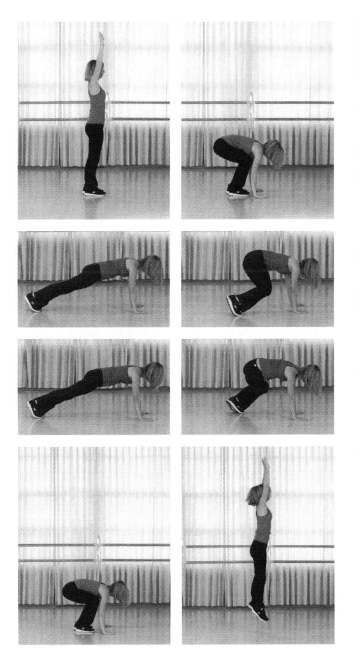

BURPEES
WITH SKI ABS

Now combine the burpee with the "Ski Abs".

Start off in a standing position with your arms extended above your head. Jump back into the plank. Then jump and bring both feet forward and to your right. Jump again and bring your feet back to the plank position. Then jump once more and bring your feet forward and to the left.

Bring your feet back to plank position. Finish by jumping forward, bringing your feet just behind your hands, and then either jumping or standing back up, with your arms straight up in the air.

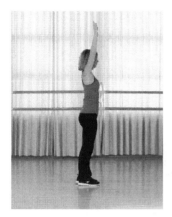
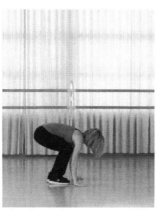
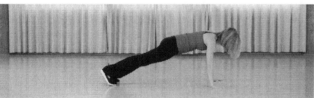
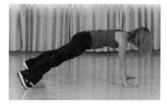
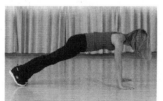
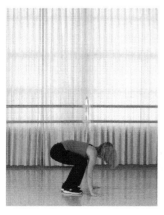
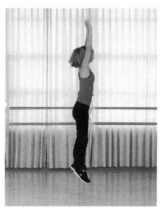

BURPEES
OPEN & CLOSE

Now combine the Burpee with the "Plank Open & Close".

Start off in a standing position with your arms extended above your head. Jump back into the plank. Then jump and bring both feet forward and to your right. Jump again and bring your feet back to the plank position.

Then jump and open your legs more than hip width apart. Quickly jump again and bring your feet together. Jump again one more time, opening your legs. Then jump again and get into the plank position.

Finish by jumping forward, bringing your feet just behind your hands, and then either jumping or standing back up, with your arms straight up in the air.

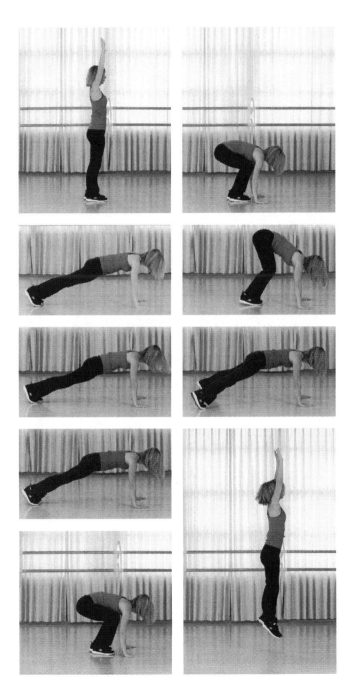

BURPEES WITH
PLANK IN & OUT
+ OPEN & CLOSE

Get into the flow with this sequence. Combine the burpees with the "Plank In & Out" and "Open & Close".

Start off in a standing position. Jump back into the plank. Then jump forward, bringing your palms just behind your palms. Jump back to the plank, and jump forward one more time.

Then jump and open your legs more than hip width apart. Quickly jump again and bring your feet together. Jump again one more time, opening your legs. Then jump again and get into the plank position.

Finish by jumping forward, bringing your feet just behind your hands, and then either jumping or standing back up, with your arms straight up in the air.

COOL DOWN

You're done! Sixteen minutes of high intensity training is up, and now you're ready to move on to stretching. I absolutely love stretching as it gives me time to let my heartbeat slow down, I help my body reduce soreness, and I get my stiff muscles to become longer. I do recommend you spend a couple of minutes cooling down after a workout.

A few stretching tips:

- Never feel pain. Stop pushing when you feel the first stretching sensation.
- Hold each stretch of a big muscle (e.g., legs) for 30 seconds. If the muscle is small (e.g., shoulders), then hold for 15 seconds.
- The first ten seconds of a stretch is the "easy stretch." After the first ten seconds, you'll get more comfortable in the stretching position, and you'll find you can push a little further.
- If you're not just looking to cool down but also want to develop flexibility, then do two sets of each stretch (or more). You will find you can go further with each set.
- Again, if you are looking for flexibility, then repeat stretching at least four times a week to get results.

If you're ready, let's stretch, release, and relax.

THE **LOWER BODY STRETCHES**

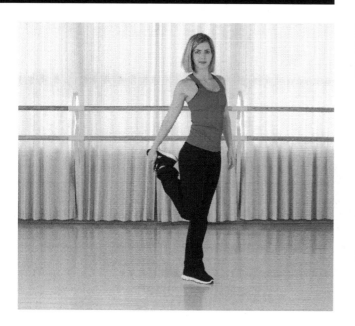

CLASSIC QUADS
STRETCH

Stand straight with your feet together. Now bend your knee, lifting your heel right next to your butt.

Catch that foot with one hand, and feel the stretch on the quads of your bent knee. Hold this position for 15 seconds and then switch legs.

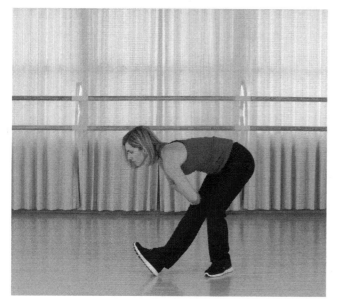

CLASSIC
HAMSTRING STRETCH

Stand straight with your feet together. Bend your back leg, and as you extend your other leg to the front, bring the heel of that leg a few inches away from your other foot.

With a straight back, bend your torso forward, feeling the stretch at the hamstrings of your extended leg. Hold this stretch for 30 seconds and then switch legs.

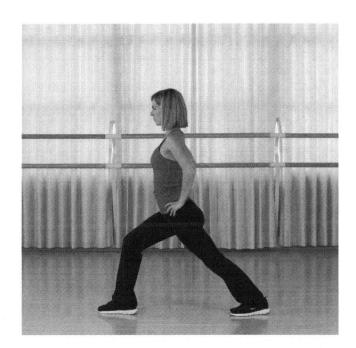

CLASSIC CALVES
STRETCH

You need this stretch—
especially after finishing a
workout with a lot of jumping
moves! Stand straight with your
feet together. Now take a rather
big step forward with one leg.
Make sure both feet point
to the front and both heels
are glued to the floor. In this
position, you should be feeling
a stretch at the calf of your back
leg. Hold it for 30 seconds, and
then switch legs. Keep your hips
square at all times.

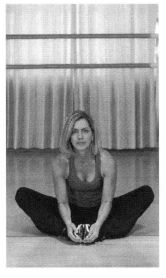

BUTTERFLY
STRETCH

Sit on the floor with your feet
against each other. Lean forward
until you feel a comfortable
stretch in your groin.
Hold for ten seconds and then
lean a little farther for a deeper
stretch. Hold for another 15
seconds.

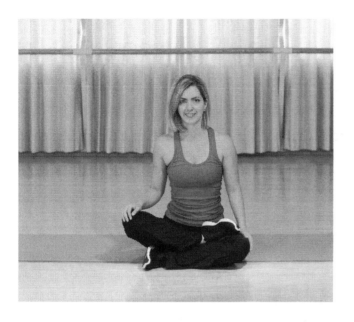

HIP STRETCH

Sit on the floor with your back straight and your knees crossed. Now lift one leg and put it on top of the other, with your upper foot on top of your lower knee. Feel the stretch in your outer thigh of your upper leg, and hold it for 15 seconds.

If this is easy, try leaning your body forward while keeping your back straight. Hold the position and once done, repeat for the other leg.

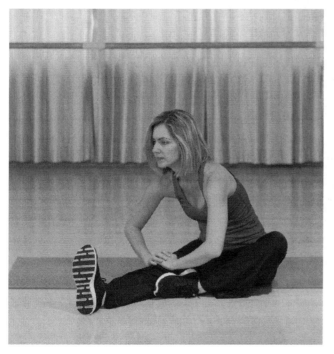

STRAIGHT-BENT
LEG STRETCH

Sit down with one leg straight and the other knee bent with the sole of the foot of the bent leg touching the inner thigh of the straight leg.

Slowly bend forward from the hips until you feel a slight stretch. Hold this position for 10 seconds. Once the tension eases up, lean a little bit more forward. Hold this position for another 20 seconds, and repeat for the other leg.

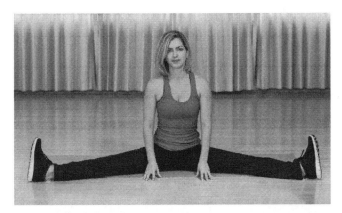

STRADDLE STRETCH

Sit down with your back straight. Open your legs a comfortable distance apart until you feel a slight stretch in your inner thighs. Hold this stretch for 10 seconds until you feel more comfortable in this position.

Then, with your back straight, place your palms on the floor in front of you and start walking your hands to the front, gradually bending your torso forward. If you can, place your elbows on the floor, and hold that stretch for 30 seconds.

Don't push yourself forward if you feel pain. You should stop and hold that position the moment you feel the stretch kicking in.

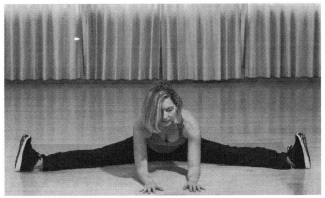

STRADDLE
HAMSTRING STRETCH

Get into the straddle stretch position. Then, with your back straight, reach toward your right leg with your left arm, stretching your right arm toward your opposite leg.

Hold this position for 30 seconds, and then repeat for other side.

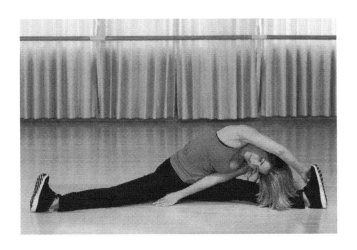

THE **UPPER BODY + CORE STRETCHES**

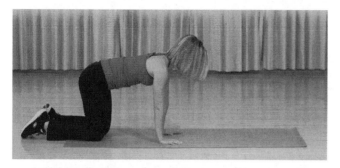

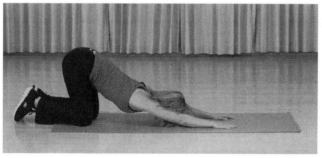

BENT BACK
STRETCH

With legs bent under you, reach forward with straight arms. Push your torso down until you feel the stretch on your back.

Hold the stretch for 15 seconds and release.

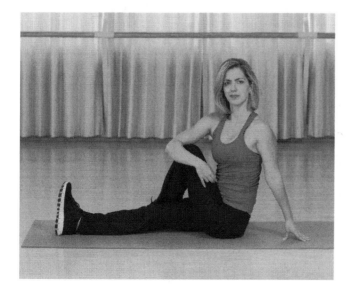

TWIST STRETCH

Sit with your right leg straight. Bend your left leg across your left foot over to the outside of your right knee. Then bend your right elbow and rest it on the outside of your left thigh.

Use your elbow to twist yourself and turn your head to look over your left shoulder. Your lower back and side hip should feel the stretch. Hold the stretch for 15 seconds, and repeat for other side.

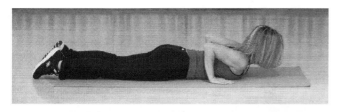

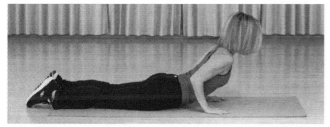

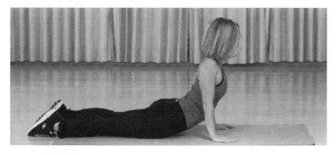

COBRA STRETCH

Lie down on the mat or on the floor, and tuck your pelvis in. Actively engage your abs. Now put your palms next to your chest and press against the floor, extending your arms while lifting your torso up and giving your abs and back a stretch.

Hold the stretch for 15 seconds and then release. Do not sink in your shoulders; instead, keep your chest lifted at all times.

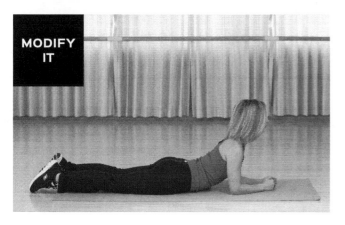

MODIFY IT

ELBOW COBRA
STRETCH

Depending on your flexibility, it might be better for you to start with the modified cobra.

Instead of having your palms almost below your shoulders, put your elbows under your shoulders, and raise your torso up. Hold the stretch for 15 seconds and then release.

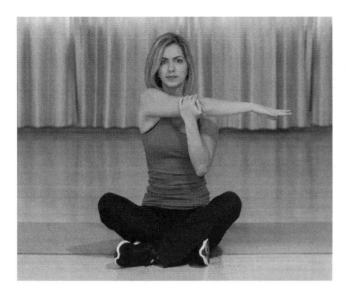

SHOULDER
STRETCH

Stand or sit straight. Pull your elbow across your chest toward your opposite shoulder. Straighten your arm, still pulling your elbow with your hand. Hold this stretch for 15 seconds and then repeat it for the other shoulder.

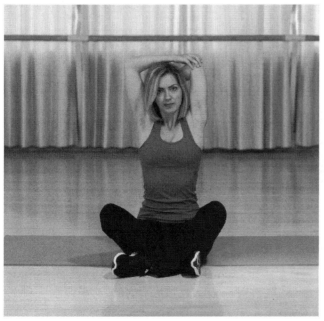

TRICEP STRETCH

Stand or sit with your back straight. Slightly bend your knees if you are standing. Bend one elbow, and put your arm behind your head. Hold your elbow with your other hand. Push your elbow to the back to stretch your shoulder and tricep (i.e., the back of your upper arm). Repeat for the other arm.

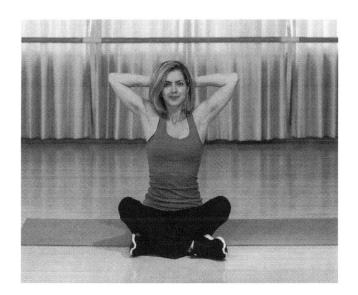

OFFICE STRETCH

Sit or stand straight. Hold the back of your head with your hands and your fingers interlaced.

Pull your shoulder blades together to create tension in your upper back and shoulders. Hold this position for 15 seconds.

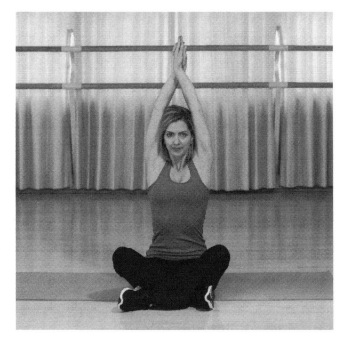

EXTENDED ARMS STRETCH

Stand or sit with your back straight. Extend your arms overhead, and cross your palms while you push your arms to the back.

Hold the stretch for 15 seconds. Switch your hand position and stretch again.

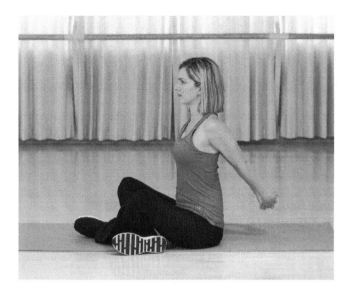

CHEST LIFT
STRETCH

This is a perfect stretch for those of us who slouch most of the day. Stand or sit with your back straight.

Bring your arms behind your back, interlace your fingers, and push your arms up, effectively lifting your chest up. Hold this stretch for 15 seconds.

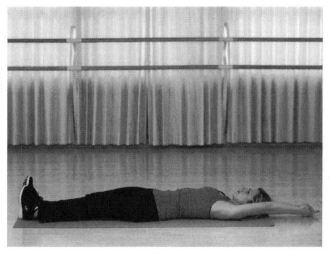

LONG BODY
STRETCH

Lie on your back with legs lengthened on the floor, arms stretched above your head, and shoulders relaxed.

Stretch your whole body, extending the tips of your fingers and toes.

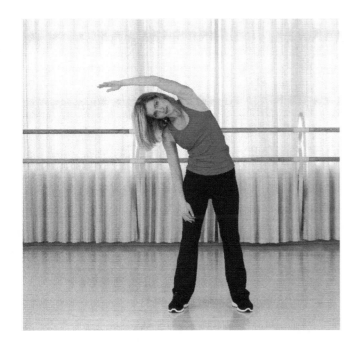

SIDE STRETCH

Stand straight with your legs hip width apart. Extend one arm up to the side of your head, palm facing the floor.

Engage your abs to hold the stretch for 15 seconds, and then repeat for the other side.

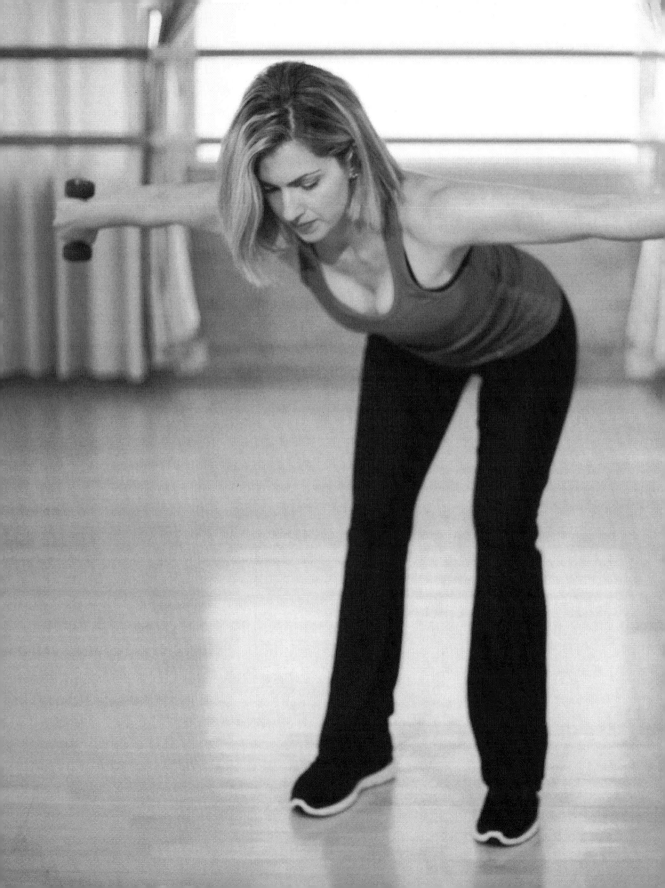

THE FB16 WORKOUT PLAN

And we're here! Ready to start exercising! For the next four weeks, you'll be exercising three times a week. In this section, we'll cover:
- How to track your progress accurately through FB16.
- How to make the best of every workout.
- How to mentally warm-up before you jump in.
- The three Blast workouts (Abs, Butt, Total Body) to follow for the next two weeks that will get you an hour's results in 16 minutes!
- And the final three Blast workouts (Balance, Upper Body, and Cardio) to do in the final two weeks of the program to get even better results!

Before you get started with exercise, take your measurements first as described in the next section. Then start exercising three times a week doing one of the Blast workouts each time. Retake those measurements once you graduate from week four. Can you see the before-after difference?

You'll find that your performance in week four will be so much better than your performance in the first week. Just try doing one of the first three workouts after you finish from week four, and see for yourself how stronger you are!

Now let's get started. Again, here are the recommended resources for this section:
- The 16-minute bonus FB16 video workout, Measurements Sheet, and Four-week Workout Calendar at:
  http://fitnessreloaded.com/fb16-book-resources/
- The FB16 interval timer at:
  http://fitnessreloaded.com/interval-timer/
- The eight-week FB16 exercise program at:
  http://fitnessreloaded.com/fb16-home-workout/

Now grab a measuring tape, and let's go.

How To Track Your Progress

In FB16 we track our progress very closely. Why? First, it's exciting to see the difference! Second, what gets measured gets better. Third, we want to have the big picture of where we stand and not just a distorted one-sided view. Let me explain.

Most people measure their progress by using the number on the scale. However, in FB16, this can be a very misleading metric. When you're exercising you are building muscle. Muscle takes less space than fat. For example, if you could hold one pound of muscle and one pound of fat, fat would have more volume than muscle. And that's why when you work out, inches might be lost, even though your weight might have not changed. If you only depend on the scale, then you won't know that you're making progress. You'll be stressing over your lack of progress without realizing you're doing awesome!

I've personally experienced this multiple times. When I got started with FB16, I felt as if I was a piece of clothing that was put in the washing machine and came out one size smaller! Even though my weight stayed the same, I had lost multiple inches from both my belly and hips.

I shrunk because I was building muscle—and burned some fat. I had less jiggly stuff going around and also developed more lean muscle. The weight on the scale stayed the same, as muscle weighs more than fat. Still, because I had built muscle and shed the jiggly stuff, my jean size dropped—and I slipped into my tightest jeans smoothly (more on this later).

And that's why in FB16 we'll be using a variety of metrics to make sure we have the whole picture of our progress in mind. What you need? A measuring tape, your tightest pants (the ones you'd like to fit into), a scale, and a camera.

The Measuring Tape Metrics
Measuring yourself with a tape will give you a much more accurate picture on whether you're shrinking or not. Before we start, go to fitnessreloaded.com/fb16-book-resources/ and download the Measurements Sheet PDF. You'll need that to track your progress throughout FB16.

Take the measuring tape, and horizontally hug your body with it as if you were a tailor. You'll be measuring three circumferences:

- Your waist, i.e., the narrowest part of your belly.
- Your belly at the belly button level
- Your hips, by placing the tape at the widest part of your hips.

Say you're measuring the circumference of your belly at the belly-button level. Place the tape right in front of your belly button and horizontally hug your body. In the Measurements Sheet, write down the number you see. That's it! Now repeat for the other two metrics.

Beware though: Make sure the tape is not extremely tight but at the same time it's not relaxed enough to fall down. Find the sweet spot where the tape feels just right. Also, it's best to take your measurements first thing in the morning, when you're less likely to be bloated.

In my opinion, the absolute best metric between these three is the hips one. The reason is that measuring your belly can sometimes lead to errors: Sometimes you're bloated. Other times you're constipated. Maybe you are into PMS mode. All three situations actively affect how big your belly is. That said you should measure all three metrics because some people may lose a lot from one body part and little from another. You need to know what's going on. When I started FB16 I immediately started losing inches from my waist. My hips followed later. If I were only measuring my hips I wouldn't have known I was actually progressing!

Okay, so you measured yourself. These are your "before" numbers. You're going to repeat those measurements four and eight weeks later. Now, even if the number on the scale doesn't change, if you are building muscle and losing fat, your measurements will reflect that.

The Jeans Test

This is by far my favorite metric! It's the most fun! You know those pants you'd like to fit into with ease, but are now too tight? Those pants that either don't go up at all, or they do get up but you need to lie down on your bed and fight with the zipper until you finish the job? Well, that's the pair of pants that qualifies for the Jeans Test.

So yes, any fabric is okay, it doesn't have to be jeans. Here's how it works. Put on your bathing suit. Now wear those pants as best as you can. Now, if they don't fit and you can only pull them up to your mid-thighs, that's all right. If you can lift them up but you cannot button them up, that's all right.

Now bring your camera. Take a picture. This is your "before" Jeans Test picture. Congrats, I'm really excited about what you'll be feeling when four weeks later you'll be comparing this picture to your "four-weeks after" picture!

You may think nothing has really changed but once you put those pictures side-by-side the difference stands out. That's the objective view of reality I want you to have.

By the way, did you notice my picture on the cover of this book? This is me wearing my tightest jeans after I graduated from the FB16 video program. At the time, if I wanted to, I could actually fit two arms inside my pants. Now these pants I had had a hard time buttoning a couple of months earlier when I was starting the program. That's the difference that happened to my own body because of FB16.

Shakira said her hips didn't lie, and your pants are not going to lie either. Even if the scale seems stuck, the pants will tell the truth. And even if you think there was not really a significant difference between your before and after photos, when you put those pictures side by side, you'll start seeing definition you had not noticed before. These changes didn't happen overnight; they happened gradually, so it's only normal to get used to them and underestimate how different your body really is. But the underestimation will be over once you put those pictures next to each other. Don't miss this opportunity to witness the change that is going to happen in your body!

Your Weight

The fact that not all changes are reflected on your scale does not mean you should not be tracking it. Again, we want to have a holistic picture. We want to be accurate. We don't want to have a distorted or subjective view of reality. And that's why we need weight too. Weigh yourself first thing in the morning and write down that number on the PDF.

The more weight you have to lose, the faster you'll see the number on the scale change. If you don't really have a lot of weight to lose, engaging in a vigorous HIIT program might not immediately show results on the scale, and if it does they'll be modest—because you didn't really have a lot to lose in the first place.

However, if you have a lot of weight to lose, the scale will still show good evidence of progress. That's not to say you shouldn't measure yourself with a tape—that's just to better set your expectations on where to look for results and how much. Stephen H. Boutcher, from the University of New South Wales in Australia, published a review article[23] in the Journal of Obesity examining the studies that have been done on HIIT and summarizing their results. He found that studies that carried out two- to six-week HIIT interventions only resulted in small 0.5–3 kg (1.1-6.6 lb.) weight loss. However, the majority of people in these short-term test studies were young adults with normal BMI and body mass.

The greatest HIIT-induced fat loss was found in two studies that used overweight type 2 diabetic adults with a BMI bigger than 29 kg/m2. The more fat you carry, the more you will lose.

So that's it about tracking your progress. Again, go to http://fitnessreloaded.com/fb16-book-resources/ to get your Measurements Sheet PDF, and you're good to go!

23 Boutcher, SH. High-Intensity Intermittent Exercise and Fat Loss. J Obes. 2011; 868305.

Make the Best of Your 16 Minutes

The top way to make the best of each 16-minute workout is to make sure you're putting your effort into it. Half-hearted effort brings half-hearted results. If you cheat and get a C for effort, you'll also get a C for results. By cheating, I mean putting less effort than what you really can put in—not (intentionally or unintentionally) changing the form of an exercise in order to make it easier. Let me explain.

There is a right and a wrong way to cheat. I know, at first it sounds crazy. Is there really a right way to cheat? The answer is yes. You're free to "cheat" when you're "modifying" an exercise to adjust it to your own fitness level. Say you're doing squats but you're not strong enough to go really low, such as at knee level. Hence, you go about three inches down, and that's it. You do what you can do. Perfect! This is the right way to "cheat."

Now, of course, you can cheat the wrong way. You can go three inches down not because you can't go lower but because you don't feel like pushing yourself. Well, you'll get the best results out of FB16 if you put your effort into it. If you don't, don't expect results to magically appear. Pretending you're exercising is not the same as actually exercising.

I understand how tempting it is to just get C for effort even though you know you could be an A+ student. I understand that when you're at home and no-body is watching over your shoulder, it's extremely tempting to wing it. But keep yourself accountable. It's only 16 minutes. You don't need to do this for long, just 16 minutes—16 minutes of your best effort.

Now, there is one more wrong way to cheat. It's meaner than the previous one. It doesn't just prevent you from getting results; it's actually harming you. Let me give you an example.

Say you want to hold the plank. So you "think" you're holding the plank, but you're actually cheating. Instead of keeping the right form, you're sticking your butt out and putting pressure on your low back in order to take it easy on your abs. That's a very common plank mistake.

We often cheat almost unconsciously when an exercise is hard, especially at first, when we haven't developed our body awareness. We ruin the form of the exercise in an effort to make it easier. Yet in our effort to make it easier, we don't just avoid exercising our muscles, we're also usually putting some other body part at risk.

If you want to make an exercise easier, do cheat, but cheat the right way. Modify the exercise to your level. Instead of holding a regular plank, hold the elbow plank, which is an easier plank variation. Instead of going low on a squat, go a little bit low. In both cases, you'll still be "cheating," but you will be doing every exercise with the right form. The right muscles will still be working, and you'll be doing it safely. The exercise will be accomplishing its purpose, and you won't be risking injury by changing the form.

Still, I'm willing to let you slack under one condition. If, say, you're at home and really tired, debating whether to work out or not, and the thought of slacking your way through your workout makes you more likely to exercise, then by all means, slack your heart out! You see, it's more important to do something rather than not do anything because you're a perfectionist. Get the difference? If you find yourself giving the "cannot try intensely enough anyway" excuse, then know that these are the weeds talking. And the weeds are trying to get you stuck where you are. Perfectionism is an unacceptable excuse in FB16, no matter how convincing it may sound. So make sure you download the FB16 calendar, and you put a check there three times a week, will ya?

Ultimately, use your common sense. Give it your best, but don't overstrain yourself. Don't push yourself if pushing yourself means sacrificing the form of the exercise. At the same time, if you get C for effort, you'll also get C for results. Know your limits, and only push up to them but not past them.

Mental Warm-Up

Before you start the workouts, let's do some mental warm-ups to ensure the best results!

You never have to be a beginner again

We usually have it the hardest when we start something new. We're like fish out of the water. We don't really know what we are doing. So if you feel like that as you're starting your workout, then keep in mind that if you keep up with FB16, then you will never have to feel like this again. You will never have to be a beginner again. So this is just a matter of you doing it and then keeping up with it. That's it.

Refrain from judgment

As you're working out, if you feel you need to stop a lot or if you feel you're not happy with your current fitness level, then I want you to refrain from judging yourself. Let me give you an analogy. I heard this one from the best-selling book *Ask and It Is Given*, and I've found it to be both effective and true. Say you want to go from Phoenix to San Diego. You really want to go to the beach. On your way to San Diego, you will have desert around you. If you look out the window as you're driving, you're only going to see desert. That's really crappy when you want to see "beach."

Yet a funny thing happens: Even though you don't see what you want to see, you still don't care! You know you're on your way to the beach. So who cares if there's desert around you now? Similarly, as you work out, give it your all, and don't judge your output, your body, or your fitness level. A few weeks from now, you will be very proud of yourself when you do this same workout and you find that it's so much easier! You will be stronger, you will be faster, and you will like exercise more—not to mention the visible results in your body. Refer to the "Remove Weeds" section should any bad thought arise. Now let's go!

Yay, you're about to get started! Use the interval timer at http://fitnessreloaded.com/interval-timer/ to help you follow through with the workouts.

ABS BLAST

Do this workout once a week, and your flat belly dreams will come true. Sixteen minutes from the start of the workout, I want you to be one step ahead. It doesn't matter if the step is big or small; what matters is progress. Don't judge yourself; give yourself time to get used to the new movements, and with time, you will just get better and better and better.

Round One (30-30 protocol)

This is your warm-up round. Take it easy. You don't need to jump as high or do too many repetitions. It's okay to go slower.

1 BOXER SHUFFLE

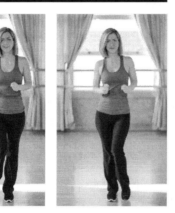

2 JOG WITH ARM ROLLS

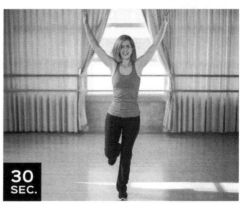

3 HIGH KNEES

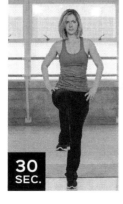
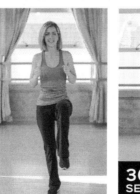

4 ALTERNATING JUMPS

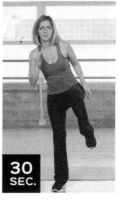
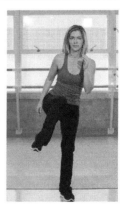

5 SHOULDER PLANK

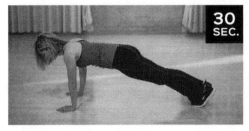

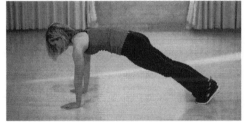

6 MOUNTAIN CLIMBERS

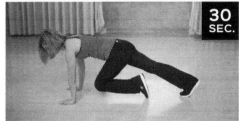

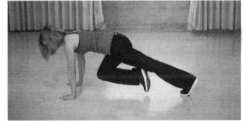

7 SCISSORS I

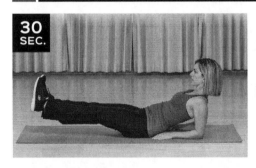

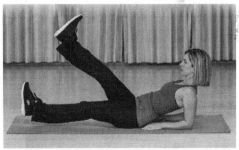

30 SEC. BREAK

Round Two (30-30 protocol)

You're warmed up now. Pick up the pace.

1 | LADYBUG

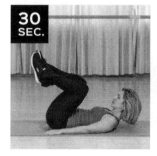
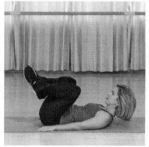
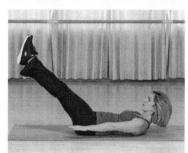

2 | ELBOW PLANK WITH HIP TWISTS

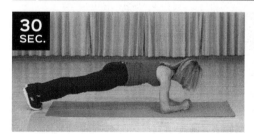
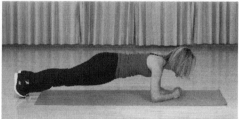

3 | PLANK WITH ALTERNATING SIDE LEG

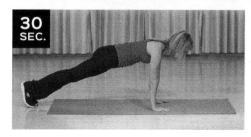
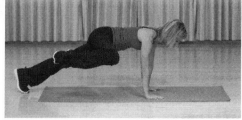

4 | C-ABS WITH STRAIGHT LEGS

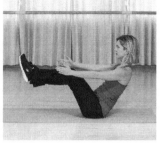
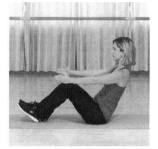
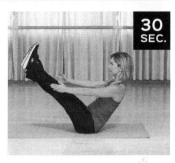

30 SEC.

5 | C-ABS OBLIQUE

30 SEC. ON EACH SIDE.

60 SEC.

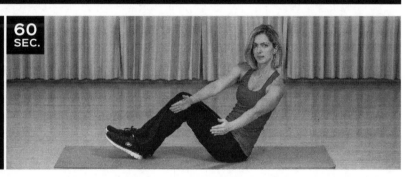

6 | FULL JUMPING BURPEES

30 SEC.

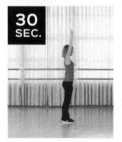
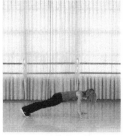
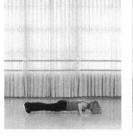
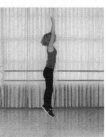

30 SEC. | BREAK

Next: Repeat Rounds One + Two

These are the final eight minutes of your workout. This is not the time to play small. This is the time to give it your all. Push yourself to go faster and do even more repetitions. This is how a strong middle is shaped.

Remember though: Never sacrifice form for speed. If you get dizzy, stop. If you ruin your form, take a break.

Cool Down

Awesome—you did it! Your abs may feel weak right now, but in the next few days, your body will be building a stronger core thanks to the work you just did today!

So now you're free to take your shower or devote another two minutes to do the following stretches:

1 | SIDE STRETCH

HOLD FOR 15 SEC. ON EACH SIDE.

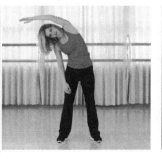

2 | CHEST LIFT STRETCH

HOLD FOR 15 SEC.

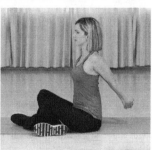

3 | COBRA STRETCH

HOLD THE STRETCH FOR 15 SEC.

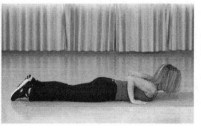
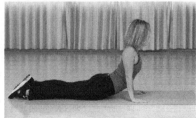

BUTT BLAST

Want a nicely shaped butt and lean legs? Maybe you want a butt that defies gravity no matter your age? You're at the right place. Let's do it.

→

Round One (20-10 protocol)

This is your warm-up round. Take it easy. It's okay to go slow.

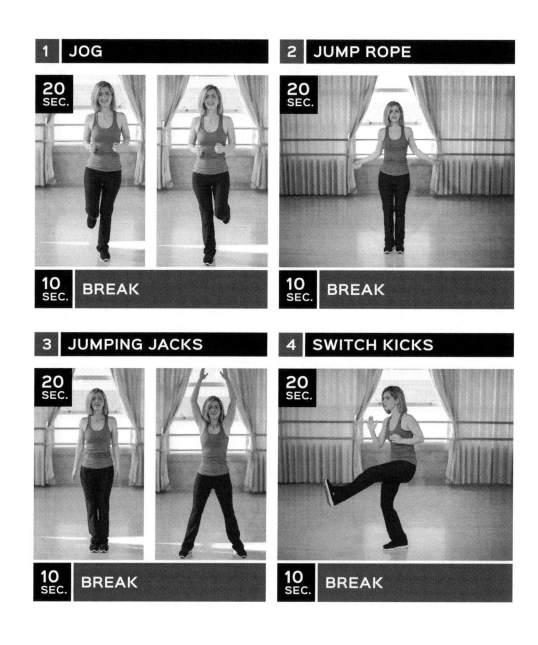

1 | JOG
20 SEC.
10 SEC. | BREAK

2 | JUMP ROPE
20 SEC.
10 SEC. | BREAK

3 | JUMPING JACKS
20 SEC.
10 SEC. | BREAK

4 | SWITCH KICKS
20 SEC.
10 SEC. | BREAK

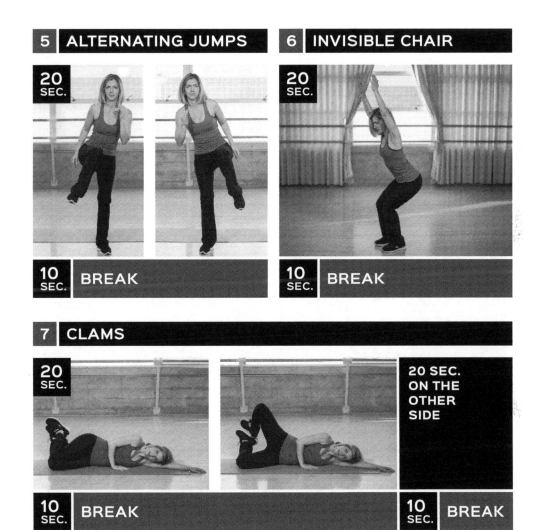

5 ALTERNATING JUMPS

20 SEC.

10 SEC. BREAK

6 INVISIBLE CHAIR

20 SEC.

10 SEC. BREAK

7 CLAMS

20 SEC.

20 SEC. ON THE OTHER SIDE

10 SEC. BREAK

10 SEC. BREAK

Round Two (20-10 protocol)

You're warmed up now. Pick up the pace.

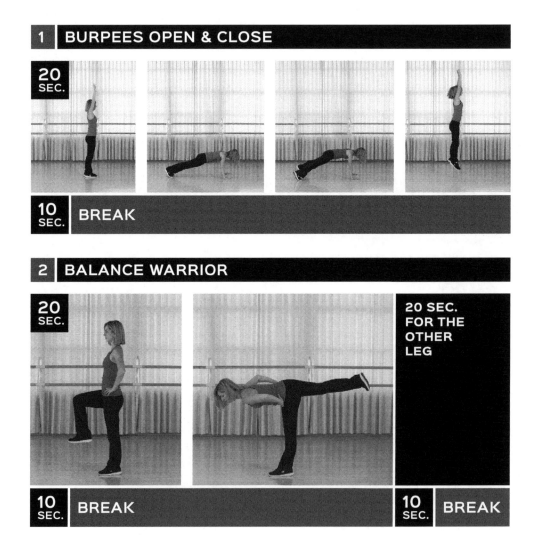

1 BURPEES OPEN & CLOSE

20 SEC.

10 SEC. BREAK

2 BALANCE WARRIOR

20 SEC.

20 SEC. FOR THE OTHER LEG

10 SEC. BREAK

10 SEC. BREAK

3 | SNOWBOARDER'S SQUATS

20 SEC.

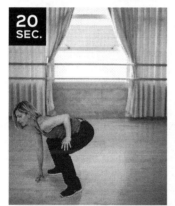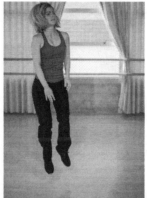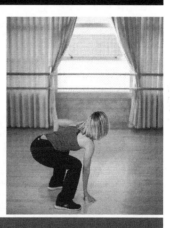

10 SEC. | BREAK

4 | SIDE ANGLE POSE

20 SEC.

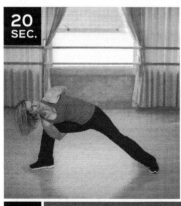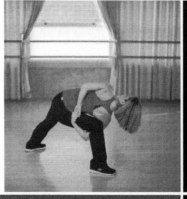

20 SEC. FOR THE OTHER LEG

10 SEC. BREAK   **10 SEC.** BREAK

5 | **REVERSE LUNGE AND KICK**

20 SEC.

20 SEC. FOR THE OTHER LEG

10 SEC. BREAK

10 SEC. BREAK

Next: Repeat Rounds One + Two

These are the final eight minutes of your workout. Give it your all. In a few weeks you'll be thinking, "Why did I find this hard? This is so easy!" As long as you put in the effort, it's not going to get harder; it's only going to get easier.

Remember though: Never sacrifice form for speed. If you get dizzy, stop. If you ruin your form, take a break.

Cool Down

Awesome—you did it! Your butt just got a lift! Starting tomorrow, the effect of gravity on your butt will be weaker.

So now you're free to take your shower or devote another two minutes to do the following stretches:

1 | BUTTERFLY STRETCH

HOLD FOR 15 SEC.

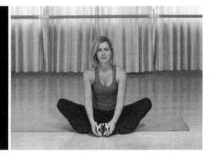 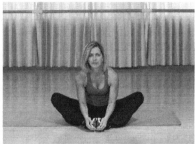

2 | STRADDLE STRETCH

HOLD FOR 30 SEC.

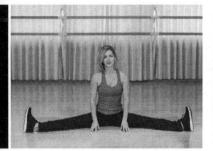 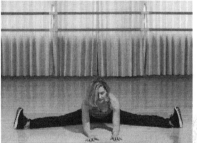

3 | STRADDLE HAMSTRING STRETCH

HOLD FOR 30 SEC. THEN REPEAT FOR THE OTHER SIDE.

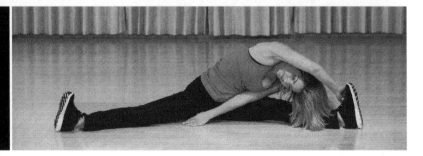

TOTAL BODY BLAST

Ready to work every inch of your body? Get your dumbbells ready. Let's do it!

Round One (30-30 protocol)

This is your warm-up round. Take it easy. It's okay to go slow.

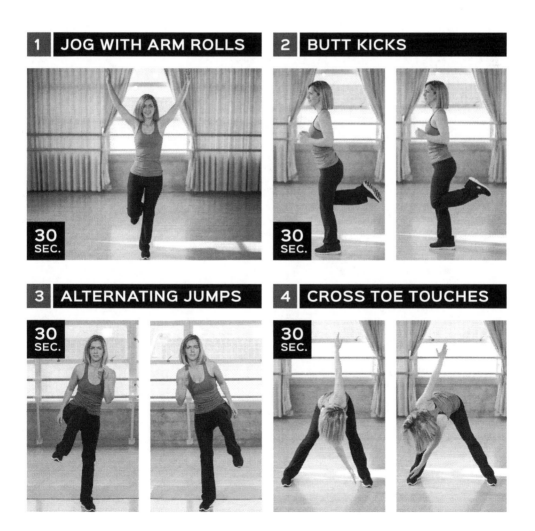

1 JOG WITH ARM ROLLS   30 SEC.

2 BUTT KICKS   30 SEC.

3 ALTERNATING JUMPS   30 SEC.

4 CROSS TOE TOUCHES   30 SEC.

5 | ARMS AND KICKS

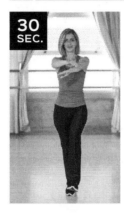 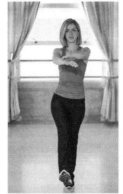

6 | KNEES AND ARMS

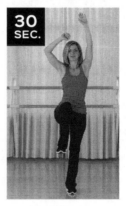 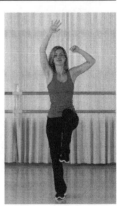

7 | SQUAT PULSES

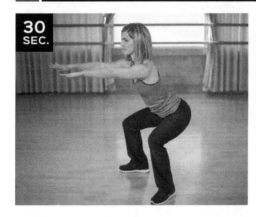 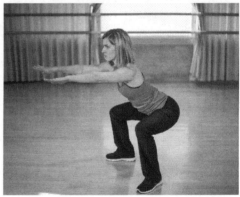

30 SEC. | BREAK

Round Two (30-30 protocol)

You're warmed up now. Pick up the pace.

1 | FULL JUMPING BURPEES

2 | BURPEES WITH SKI ABS

3 | TRICEP DIPS

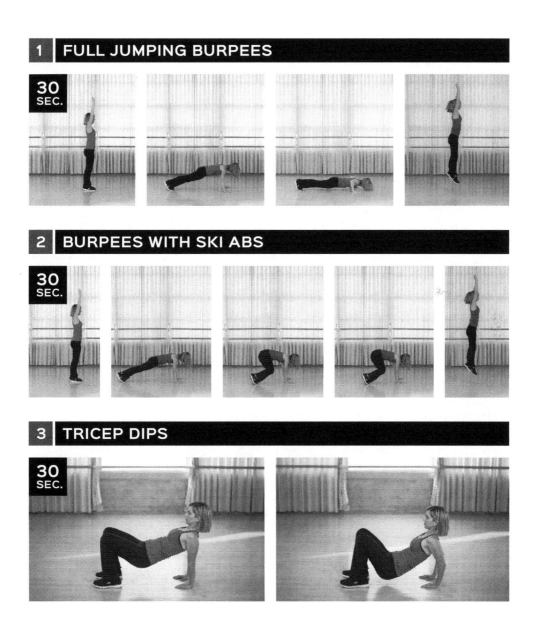

4 | BICEP CURLS ON HALF SQUAT

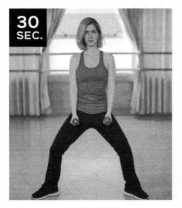
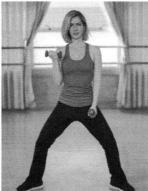
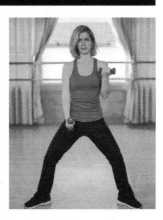

5 | ELBOW OBLIQUE CAN-CAN

30 SEC. ON EACH SIDE.

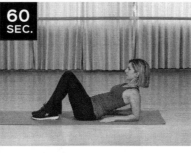
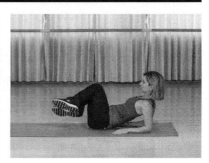
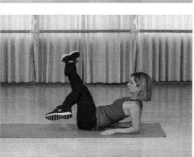
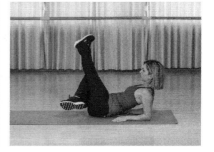

6 | SHOULDER LATERAL LIFTS

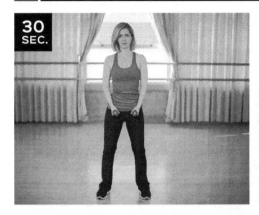 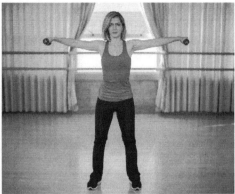

30 SEC. BREAK

Next: Repeat Rounds One + Two

Wow! You're already 50% done! Time flies! Now let's repeat those two rounds one more time—just give it your all this time. You're all warmed up; there are no excuses. It's only eight minutes. Show yourself what you can do!

Remember though: Never sacrifice form for speed. If you get dizzy, stop. If you ruin your form, take a break.

Cool Down

Woo hoo! You're done. Not everyone is doing it, but you are. You deserve a big pat on the back for this.

Let's move on to showering, or if you can spare a couple of minutes, stretching.

1 | TWIST STRETCH

HOLD FOR 15 SEC. THEN REPEAT FOR THE OTHER SIDE.

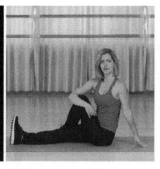

2 | TRICEP STRETCH

HOLD FOR 15 SEC. THEN REPEAT FOR THE OTHER ARM.

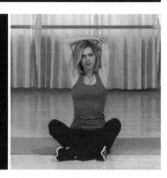

3 | SHOULDER STRETCH

HOLD FOR 15 SEC. THEN REPEAT FOR THE OTHER SHOULDER.

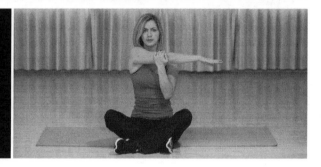

4 | CLASSIC CALVES STRETCH

HOLD FOR 30 SEC. THEN REPEAT FOR THE OTHER LEG.

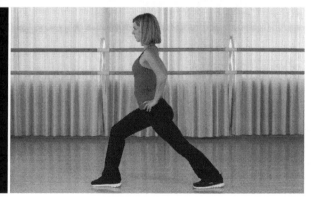

THE WORKOUTS: **WEEKS THREE AND FOUR**

Ok, you're now ready to step it up. Your first two weeks helped you adjust to the new intensity level. Now it's time to experiment with more exercises, and get to the next level. Let's do it!

BALANCE BLAST

Whenever I think of the word "balance," I think about work-life balance. Well, FB16, being efficient and effective, definitely assists you with that balance as well. Now let's work on our neuromotor balance skills while at the same time getting an awesome workout!

$\rightarrow$

Round One (20-10 protocol)

This is your warm-up round. Take it easy. It's okay to go slow.

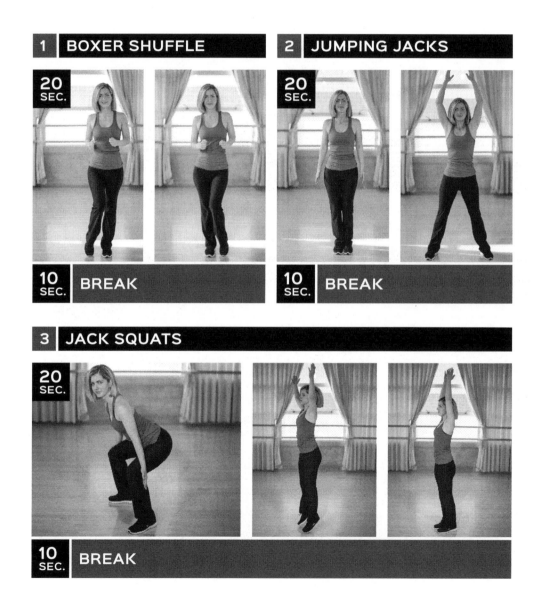

4 | SPRINTER'S SQUAT

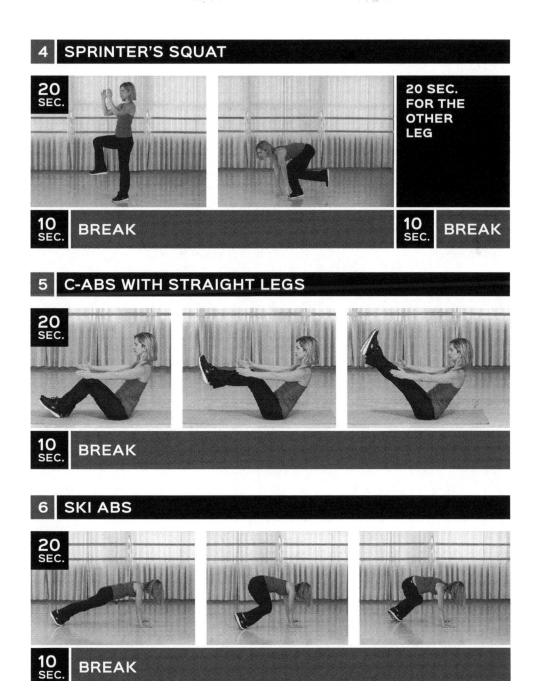

20 SEC.

20 SEC. FOR THE OTHER LEG

10 SEC. | BREAK

10 SEC. | BREAK

5 | C-ABS WITH STRAIGHT LEGS

20 SEC.

10 SEC. | BREAK

6 | SKI ABS

20 SEC.

10 SEC. | BREAK

7 | DIAMOND JUMPS

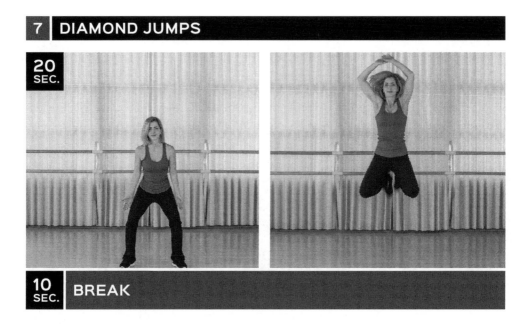

20 SEC.

10 SEC. | BREAK

Round Two (20-10 protocol)

You're warmed up now. Pick up the pace.

1 JUMPING LUNGES

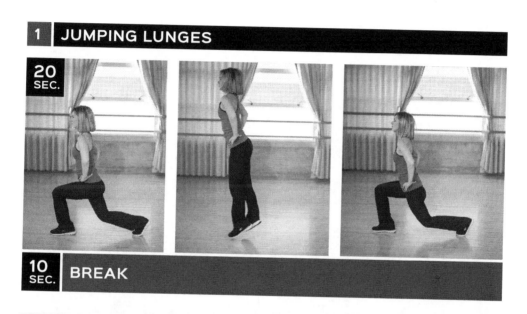

20 SEC.

10 SEC. BREAK

2 SQUAT AND SIDE LEG STRAIGHT

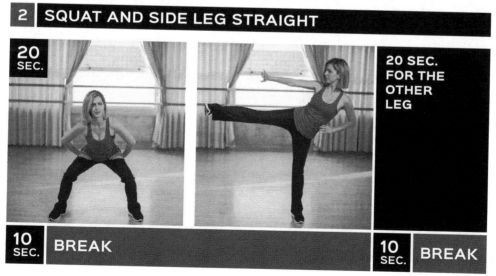

20 SEC.

20 SEC. FOR THE OTHER LEG

10 SEC. BREAK

10 SEC. BREAK

3 | PLANK WITH ARM UP

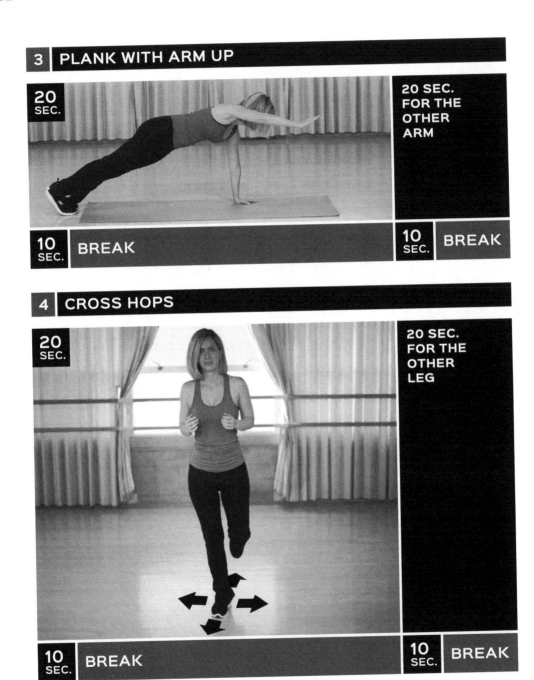

20 SEC.

20 SEC. FOR THE OTHER ARM

10 SEC. BREAK

10 SEC. BREAK

4 | CROSS HOPS

20 SEC.

20 SEC. FOR THE OTHER LEG

10 SEC. BREAK

10 SEC. BREAK

5 | SHOULDER BRIDGE ON TOES

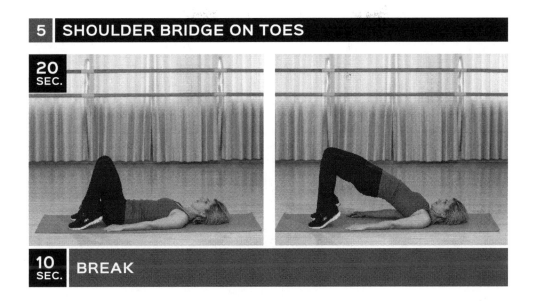

20 SEC.

10 SEC. BREAK

Next: Repeat Rounds One + Two

Almost done! Now that you've tried these exercises once, it's going to be easier next time. Let's do it!

Remember: Never sacrifice form for speed. If you get dizzy, stop. If you ruin your form, take a break.

Cool Down

Wonderful, you're all done. And you're now able to balance just a little bit better than you could 16 minutes ago. Now let's take a shower. If you're not in a hurry, let's do some stretching. Here are my recommendations:

1	HIP STRETCH

HOLD FOR 30 SEC.

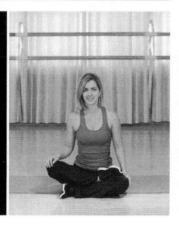

2	STRADDLE STRETCH

HOLD FOR 30 SEC.

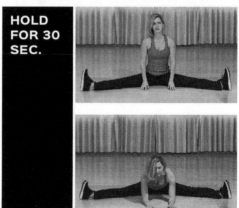

3	STRAIGHT-BENT LEG STRETCH

HOLD FOR 30 SEC. THEN REPEAT FOR THE OTHER LEG.

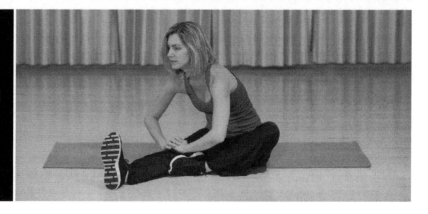

UPPER BODY BLAST

Men find working on their upper body easier than women. I know my husband is just so much better at push-ups than I am! But that's just one more reason to work on my upper body strength—which is exactly what we'll be doing today. Get your dumbbells, and let's get started.

→

Round One (20-10 protocol)

This is your warm-up round. Take it easy. It's okay to go slow.

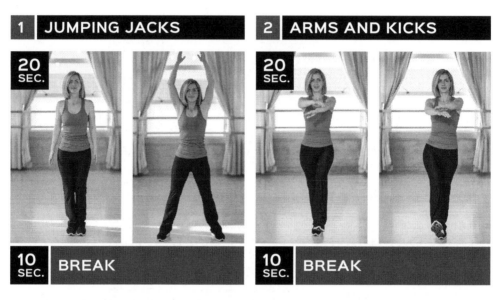

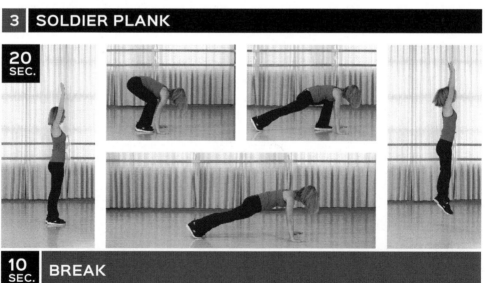

4 | ARM WINGS

20 SEC.

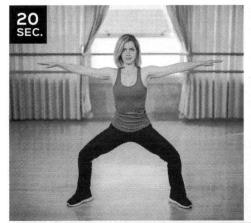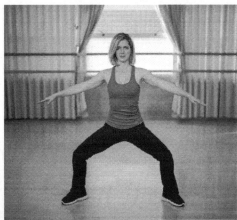

10 SEC. BREAK

5 | BICEP CURLS ON HALF SQUAT

20 SEC.

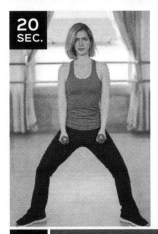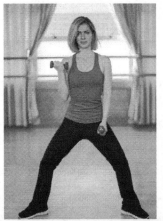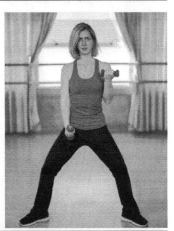

10 SEC. BREAK

6 | HAMMERS ON HALF SQUAT

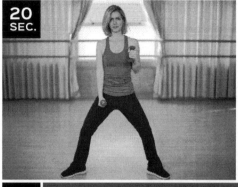
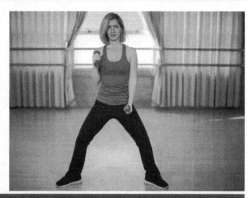

20 SEC.

10 SEC. | BREAK

7 | SCARECROWS

8 | ROWS

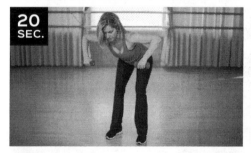
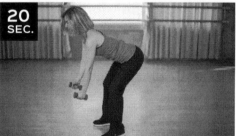

20 SEC.

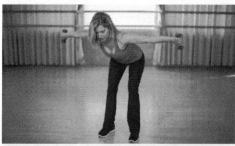
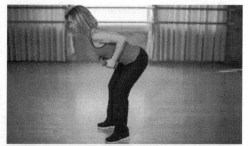

10 SEC. | BREAK

10 SEC. | BREAK

Round Two (20-10 protocol)

You're warmed up now. Pick up the pace.

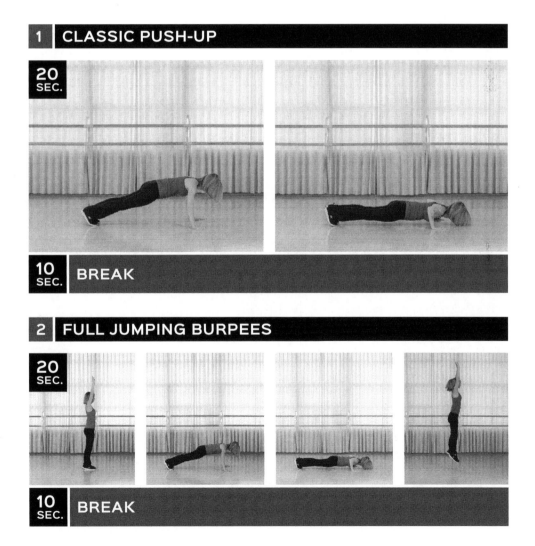

1 | CLASSIC PUSH-UP

20 SEC.

10 SEC. | BREAK

2 | FULL JUMPING BURPEES

20 SEC.

10 SEC. | BREAK

3 BURPEES WITH MOUNTAIN CLIMBERS

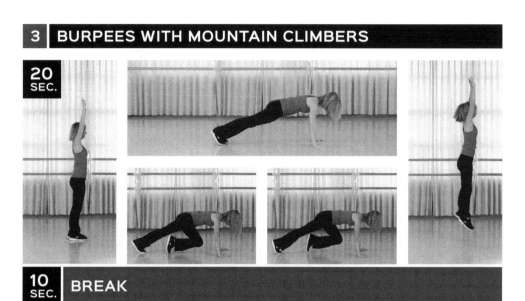

20 SEC.

10 SEC. BREAK

4 TRICEP CAN-CAN

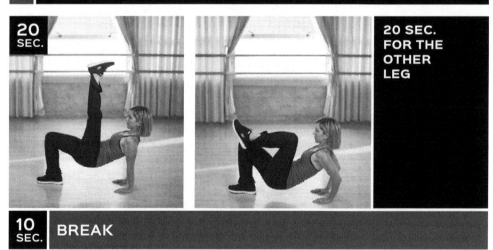

20 SEC.

20 SEC. FOR THE OTHER LEG

10 SEC. BREAK

5 | WIDER SHOULDER PULSES

20 SEC.

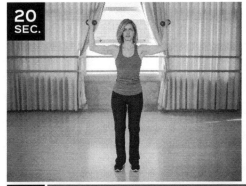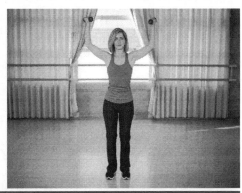

10 SEC. BREAK

6 | SHOULDER PULSES

20 SEC.

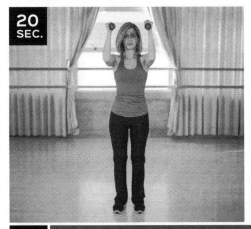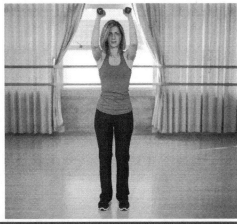

10 SEC. BREAK

7 | SHOULDER LATERAL LIFTS

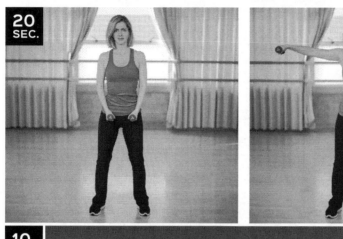

20 SEC.

10 SEC. BREAK

Next: Repeat Rounds One + Two

Whoa, already halfway to the end! How has it been so far? Now, these are the final eight minutes of your workout. Give it your all.

Remember: Never sacrifice form for speed. If you get dizzy, stop. If you ruin your form, take a break.

Cool Down

Yeah, lean arms and back! This is exactly how they are built. Congratulations on finishing one more workout! You're free to take your shower or devote another two minutes for stretching.

1 | BENT BACK STRETCH

HOLD FOR 15 SEC.

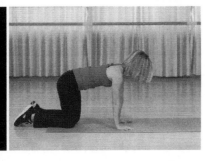
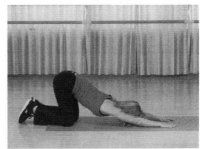

2 | EXTENDED ARMS STRETCH

HOLD FOR 15 SEC. AND THEN SWITCH YOUR HAND POSITION AND RE-PEAT

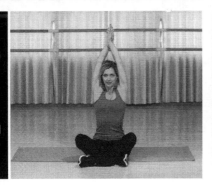
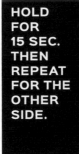

3 | TRICEP STRETCH

HOLD FOR 15 SEC. THEN REPEAT FOR THE OTHER SIDE.

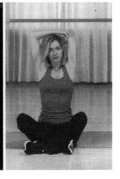

CARDIO BLAST

I believe this is the hardest workout included in this book. I know some people don't want me to "warn" them in advance—they say I lower their motivation. But that's not what I want. Instead, I want you to be prepared. If you find yourself out of breath, it's comforting to know that this is indeed a hard workout and that it's normal to be exhausted.

Cardio Blast is definitely the most calorie-burning workout of this book as it includes almost non-stop cardio with jumping and leg exercises sprinkled throughout. Now bring a chair, and let's burn the saddlebacks, the muffin top, or whatever it is you want to get rid of!

Round One (30-30 protocol)

This is your warm-up round. Take it easy. It's okay to go slow.

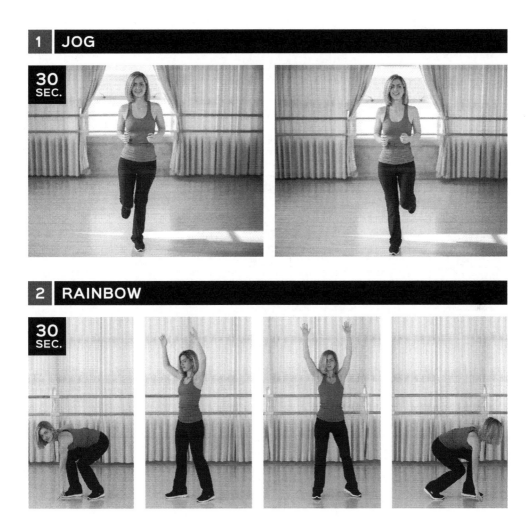

3 | HIGH KNEES

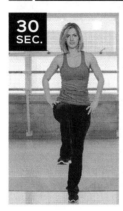
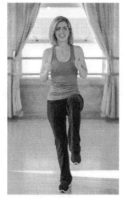

4 | KNEES AND ARMS

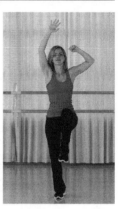
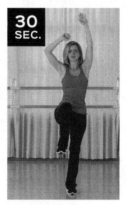

5 | SIDE STEPS

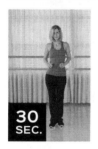
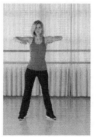
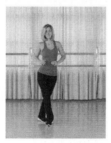
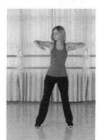
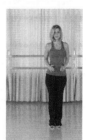

6 | ALTERNATING LUNGES

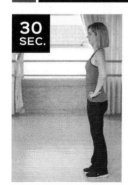
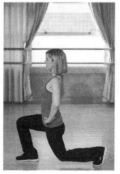
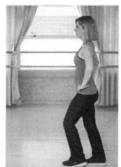
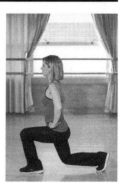

7 | TABLE KICKS

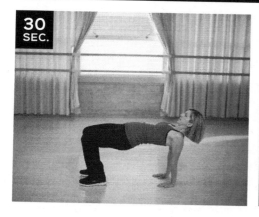 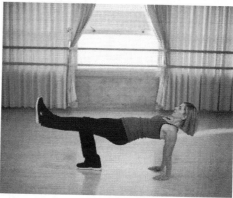

30 SEC. | **BREAK**

Round Two (30-30 protocol)
You're warmed up now. Pick up the pace.

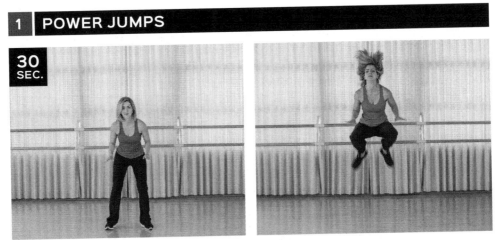

1 POWER JUMPS

30 SEC.

2 CHAIR SIDE LIFTS

30 SEC. FOR EACH LEG.

60 SEC.

3 | JACK SQUATS

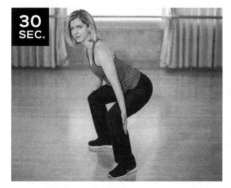
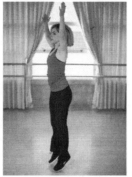
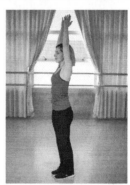

30 SEC.

4 | CHAIR LUNGES

30 SEC. FOR EACH LEG.

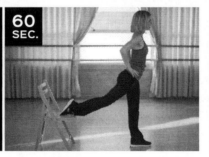
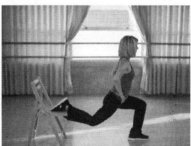

60 SEC.

5 | SKI JUMPS

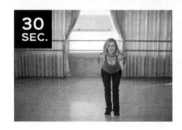
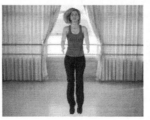
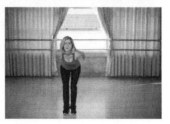

30 SEC.

30 SEC. BREAK

Next: Repeat Rounds One + Two

Did I say congratulations for doing the final workout of this book? Oh I'm sorry, my bad—big congrats to you for sticking with FB16! Now, another eight minutes left; the workout will be over, while you will be leaner! Sounds like a good deal to me!

Remember: Never sacrifice form for speed. If you get dizzy, stop. If you ruin your form, take a break.

Cool Down

This is a much-needed cool down after 16 minutes of the Cardio Blast! I strongly recommend you spend a few minutes cooling down and getting your heart rate down. Let's do some stretching:

1 CLASSIC QUADS STRETCH

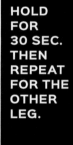

HOLD
FOR
30 SEC.
THEN
REPEAT
FOR THE
OTHER
LEG.

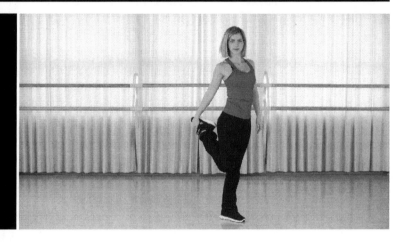

2 | CLASSIC HAMSTRING STRETCH

HOLD
FOR
30 SEC.
THEN
REPEAT
FOR THE
OTHER
LEG.

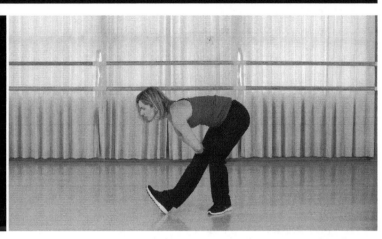

3 | BENT BACK STRETCH

HOLD
FOR
30 SEC.

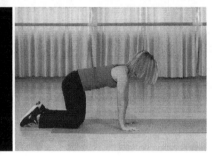

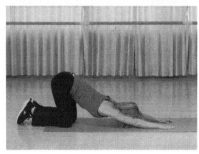

Beyond the Four Week Program

You're done with the four week Program! Now what? First, take your "After" picture! The Jeans Test is very important. Even if you think nothing has changed, the pictures will prove you wrong once you put them side-by-side. Just try it. Don't be lazy with documenting your progress.

Second, use the tape to take your "after" measurements and jot them down on your measurements PDF. What's the difference? I'm curious!

But what about exercise, you may ask. Here are my recommendations:

- This book contains more than 100 exercises. Time to create your own workouts?
- Repeat the workouts of this book for one more month, making it an eight-week program.
- Advanced exercisers only: Repeat the workouts of this book for one more month, yet doubling them this time. For example, this would mean you'd do the Abs and the Butt Blasts together, effectively creating a 32-minute workout. Doubling the workouts is not for everyone, but if you're passionate about exercise and want to see even greater results, then give it a try.
- Join the eight-week video program at http://fitnessreloaded.com/fb16-home-workout/ and come work out with me!
- And don't forget about your bonus 16-minute workout at http://fitnessreloaded.com/fb16-book-resources/.

Let me just congratulate you once again for following through. Persistence is the key to success, and you got this! I'm really proud for you. Do contact me at http://fitnessreloaded.com/contact/ and tell me your results, or send me your Jeans Test Before—After pictures! I can't wait to find out what happened!

EPILOGUE

"Why are these people working out?!" I'd ask my mom with surprise when I'd see tourists exercising at the five-star hotel's fitness center. I was nine years old, and I was vacationing with my family at a hotel in Greece. Seeing those "foreigners" working out at the gym just didn't make sense. Obelix, Asterix's best friend, would say: "These Romans are crazy!" Just like him, I'd think, "These tourists are crazy!" My rationale was that when on vacation, you're not supposed to work. That's the very definition of vacation! So why were these people working? My mom had answered that these "foreigners" had a different (better) culture than the Greeks and that exercise was a lifestyle for them. I'd still find it so out of the ordinary. No Greek would ever go to the hotel's gym when on vacation!

I now understand why they were at the gym. I understand that when you're used to working out, your body is literally asking for it. Just like you don't take a vacation from "food," "water," or "peeing," you also don't want to take a vacation from exercise.

A lot has changed since then. Exercise is now part of my lifestyle. I enjoy it. I feel as if something is missing if I don't do it. But the change took time. Just a couple of years ago, when I'd see people doing really intense exercise, I'd cringe. I would have never tried doing something that gets me that sweaty and requires that much effort. Yes, I did exercise, but I preferred "easy-going" exercise that was not as challenging.

I now no longer have that fear. I actually enjoy the challenge! Really! Can you believe it? Well, of course you can—you just read my book! But when I ponder about the extent to which I have changed, sometimes it still feels that this is not me!

But it is me! This is just one of those cases where you change unexpectedly.

Have you ever done anything that was so different than what you'd normally do that you surprised yourself? Maybe you didn't expect to have kids, and boom, that baby was born. You're a mom! Or you didn't expect to like that job, and you got hooked. Or you got really successful at work, and you're still pinching yourself that this actually happened!

This is all evidence that things you may consider impossible may actually be possible. This is the end of this book but the start of a new journey. Even if you've done high intensity training before, you're on a different path now. You now have more clarity about what you want. You have more clarity on what you like versus what you don't like. You're at a better place and can make better decisions. You have one more resource in your toolbox to feel better, look better, and live the life you really want to live.

Are you excited? It's all a matter of time before you see more and more good changes coming to your life! Believe it, commit to it, and it's inevitable. Nobody will be able to stop those changes from happening. You'll be unstoppable! Enjoy the journey!

About the Author

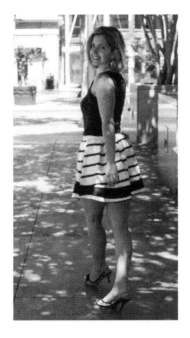

Born and raised in the island of Crete in Greece, best-selling author Maria Brilaki is a Stanford Engineering grad with an MBA. She founded Fitness Reloaded in 2011 to inspire busy professionals live a full life–enjoy worldly success while also being in amazing shape, having great energy, and enjoying every minute.

Maria was not always a healthy living advocate. Yet after experiencing the insidious weight gain and energy leaks that come with an office job, she decided to change direction and make living a long, vital life a chief aspiration.

Yet, she didn't want to live healthier the way most people she knew were going about it–through endless restriction and sheer force. She felt she *had* to put her brains into finding alternative, more effective, and at the same time pleasurable ways to do it.

Her approach worked. Maria eats whatever she wants, including the–lately vilified–carbs. She also does not work out all day, just enough so that her body feels satisfied and nourished. She enjoys life and takes care of her body because it feels good to do it, not out of duty.

Maria lives with her husband in sunny and ambitious Silicon Valley in California. She religiously spends part of every summer enjoying the crystal blue Greek beaches.

Her work has already helped more than 50,000 people change their health habits. *Flat Belly, Firm Butt in 16 Minutes* is her second book. Maria has not even turned thirty.

Acknowledgements

I'd like to thank the people who have assisted me with the creation of the FB16 program and the writing of this book.

First, I want to thank my husband Christos. He provides me with the support and stability I need to be my most creative self.

Second, I want to thank all the pilot students of the eight-week FB16 program. They were the ones who did it first, and their feedback was instrumental in the development of the final program. Special thanks to (in no particular order): Sarah, Jessica, Dayna, Gaelle, Helen T., Helen Z., Lexi, Kelly, Donna, Charlotte, Amanda, Melanie, Aleks, Yev, Vicky, Claudia, Krista, Stephanie, Janice, Eleana, Anja, Stacia, and Marcela.

Next, I want to thank the people who have made FB16—this dream of mine—come true: the amazing designer, Maria Gratsia; Nick Testa, the photographer and videographer; Anna Vassiliadis, the "savior" video editor; John Karpouchtsis, the nicest ever web developer; Emmanuel Lucio, whose research skills came in handy; Daphne Parsekian, the book editor; and Mary Sano, who provided her dance studio for the FB16 shots.

I also want to thank all my Facebook friends, who happily voiced their opinions and helped Maria and me create an amazing book cover.

Finally, I want to thank the people who kindly reviewed this book: Pauline Cheung and Helen Thornber.

INDEX